ClinLab Navigator's

Essentials of Transfusion Medicine

First Edition
2008

Frederick V. Plapp, MD, PhD

ClinLab Navigator's Essentials of Transfusion Medicine

ISBN-10: 1-4196-5661-9

Copyright © 2008 by ClinLab Navigator, LLC.

Managing Editor Chris V. Plapp

Design and Layout by Collin A. Harbison

NOTICE

As new scientific information becomes available through basic and clinical research, recommended treatments and drug therapies undergo changes. The author(s) and publisher have done everything possible to make this book accurate, up to date and in accord with accepted transfusion medicine standards at the time of publication. To the fullest extent of the law, neither the authors nor the publisher assumes any liability for any injury and/or damage to persons or property arising out of or related to any use of material contained in this book. Any practice described in this book should be applied by the reader in accordance with professional standards of care used in regard to the unique circumstances that may apply in each situation. Readers are advised to check the most current information provided on procedures featured or by the manufacturer of each product to be administered, to verify the recommended dose or formula, the method and duration of administration, and contraindications. It is the responsibility of the practitioner, relying on their own experience and knowledge of the patient, to make diagnoses, to determine dosages and the best treatment for each individual patient, and to take all appropriate safety precautions.

The most up to date information can always be found on our web site
(http://www.clinlabnavigator.com).

Preface

This book is intended to be a readily accessible compendium of the information needed to practice transfusion medicine on a daily basis in a hospital setting.

References were not included in the text, but are available by contacting the author through ClinLabNavigator.com.

Frederick V. Plapp, MD PhD

Medical Director

Saint Luke's Regional Laboratories

Saint Luke's Hospital

Kansas City, MO 64111

Medical Director of ClinLabNavigator.com

This book is dedicated to Drs. Masahiro Chiga, David C. Jenkins, and Richard T. O'Kell. These three mentors were most influential in inspiring me to immerse myself in clinical pathology and transfusion medicine.

CHAPTER 1:
Blood Group Antigens and Antibodies

BLOOD GROUP SYSTEM GENETICS

A blood group system includes those antigens that are produced by alleles at a single genetic locus on a chromosome or those produced by alleles at loci that are so closely linked that crossing-over between them either does not occur or is extremely rare. The alternative genes at a single locus are termed alleles and are said to be antithetical to each other. In a majority of blood group systems the same term is used to describe the blood group gene and the antigen whose production it controls. In order to indicate whether gene or antigen is intended, gene symbols are set in italics or are underlined. Thus, the *M* gene codes for production of M antigen, the *Jkᵃ* gene for production of the Jkᵃ antigen. Most blood group genes are autosomal and co-dominant; inherited traits are expressed whether the allele is present in the homozygous or heterozygous form. A few produce no detectable antigen and are termed amorphs.

The antigen is the structure on the red cell membrane that is able to complex with its specific antibody. A phenotype is a description of which antigens are present on an individual's red cells whereas a genotype is a description of an individual's genes. Phenotypes are determined by serological tests that reveal the presence or absence of antigens on red cells. Genotypes can only be determined definitively by family studies and DNA genotyping.

An individual who has identical genes at a given locus on both paired chromosomes is homozygous at that locus whereas, if different genes are present, the individual is heterozygous.

THE ABO BLOOD GROUP SYSTEM

The most important blood group system is the ABO system. ABO antigens are carbohydrates. There are three alleles at the ABO locus on the long arm of chromosome 9: A, B and O. The A gene results in the expression of A antigen on the red cells and the B gene results in the expression of B antigen. The O gene does not produce a detectable blood group antigen.

The *A* gene codes for production of a galactosaminyl transferase that adds N-acetylgalactosamine to a precursor carbohydrate chain bearing H antigen. The *B* gene codes for production of a galactosyl transferase that adds D-galactose to the same H-bearing chain. The *O* gene is similar to A except for a single base deletion which shifts the reading frame. As a result, the O gene does not make a functional transferase and Group O cells express only H antigen.

The H antigen is produced by a fucosyl transferase coded for by the *H* gene on Chromosome 19. Individuals who inherit two *h* genes (*h* being a rare amorphic allele of *H*) cannot add A, B or H immunodominant sugars to the precursor chain and appear group O. This rare phenotype is known as the Bombay or O_h phenotype. Individuals with the Bombay phenotype can make potent antibodies to A, B and H and are compatible only with red cells from other Bombay individuals.

The following table summarizes the antigens and antibodies of the ABO blood group system.

ABO Antigens and Antibodies

Group	RBC Antigen	Genotypes	Plasma Antibodies
O	-	O/O	Anti-A & - B
A	A	A/O, A/A	Anti-B
B	B	B/O, B/B	Anti-A
AB	A, B	A/B	-

As seen in the table, phenotype A can be produced by genotype AA or AO. Group A can be further subdivided into A_1 and A_2.

The frequency of ABO blood groups differs in various ethnic populations, as seen in the following table. African Americans are more likely to have group B phenotype compared to Caucasians.

ABO blood groups in different U.S. populations

ABO Group	Caucasian American	African American	Asian American	Native American
O	45	49	40	79
A	40	27	28	16
B	11	20	27	4
AB	4	4	5	<1

Individuals who lack the A antigen on their red cells have anti-A in their plasma and those who lack the B antigen have anti-B. These are primarily IgM antibodies and are termed naturally occurring or expected antibodies because they develop in all individuals even in the absence of a known antigenic stimulus. In contrast, most other red cell antibodies are IgG antibodies and develop as a result of an immune response following transfusion or pregnancy. They are termed immune or unexpected antibodies.

One must not transfuse red cells that contain A and/or B antigen to an individual with the corresponding antibody since these antibodies cause hemolysis. Transfusing incompatible plasma (e.g. group O plasma to a group A individual) is also generally avoided but is not as critical because incompatible plasma is quickly diluted with the much larger plasma volume of the recipient. However, hemolysis can occur with transfusion of large volumes of plasma or transfusion of plasma with exceptionally potent antibodies.

THE RH BLOOD GROUP SYSTEM

The Rh blood group system is the second most important system and is the most complex. It is important because it is associated with hemolytic transfusion reactions and with development of severe hemolytic disease of the newborn (HDN). Rh antigens are proteolipids and lack carbohydrate.

The inheritance of Rh antigens is determined by a complex of 2 closely linked genes on chromosome 1. One gene codes for the protein carrying D expression; the other codes for the proteins carrying C or c and E or e expression. Rh-positive individuals have both a *D* and a *CE* gene while Rh-negative individuals have only a *CE* gene. Depending on which genes are present on a chromosome, 8 common antigen combinations or haplotypes are possible: Dce, DCe, DcE, DCE, dce, dCe, dcE, and dCE. Common phenotypes and genotypes are given below.

D antigen is the most important Rh antigen. Presence of a single D antigen confers upon an individual the designation Rh-positive; its absence means that the person is Rh-negative. Eighty five percent of Caucasians, 92% of African Americans and 99% of Asian Americans are Rh positive. The letter d is commonly used to indicate the lack of D in Rh-negative individuals, but neither d antigen nor anti-d has been detected.

The Fisher-Race nomenclature has been more widely adopted over the more complex Wiener nomenclature for Rh antigens. However, an abbreviated version of the Wiener system is useful to describe Rh genotypes. Wiener is convenient because it uses a single letter, R or r, with superscripts to name a 3 locus haplotype. It is possible to translate from one nomenclature to the other by remembering a few rules:

- In the Wiener system, D is indicated by an uppercase R and the absence of D is indicated by lower case r.

- In the Wiener system, superscripts or numbers are used to indicate which Cc or Ee genes are present. Numbers are used with R and primes are used with r.

- In the Fisher Race system, loci are lined up in the order Dd, Cc, Ee (e.g. DCE)

- In the Wiener system, the Dd position is numbered 0, Cc position is 1 and Ee position is 2.

- The Wiener superscript of 0, 1, 2 indicates which of the Fisher Race loci is in its uppercase form (D, C, or E). For example, 1 or prime indicates that C is capitalized, while a 2 or double prime indicates that E is capitalized.

Rh Nomenclature and Haplotype Frequencies

Fisher Race	Wiener	% Caucasians	% African Americans	% Asian Americans
Dce	R^0	4	44	3
DCe	R^1	42	17	70
DcE	R^2	14	11	21
DCE	R^z	0.2	0	1
dce	r	37	26	3
dCe	r'	2	2	2
dcE	r''	1	0	0
dCE	r^y	0	0	0

The most common haplotype in Caucasians and Asian Americans is DCe (R^1), while the most common phenotype in African Americans is Dce (R^0). Red blood cells that fail to react with all Rh antibodies are called Rh null. An individual's genotype can only be determined with certainty by performing DNA analysis and family studies.

Unlike the ABO naturally occurring antibodies, Rh antibodies are produced in response to an incompatible transfusion or pregnancy. The D antigen is the most immunogenic of the Rh antigens, causing immunization at least 50% of the time when a D-negative person receives a single unit of D-positive blood. Anti-c is the second most important Rh antibody. Although anti-E is more common than anti-c, anti-E is frequently a naturally occurring antibody. Anti-c and anti-e only occur after an antigenic stimulus. Antibodies to Rh antigens are primarily IgG antibodies which can cross the placenta and hemolyze the red cells of the fetus, resulting in HDN.

OTHER BLOOD GROUP SYSTEMS

More than 400 other blood group antigens exist. Even though blood is ABO and Rh compatible, a recipient of a transfusion may still develop an alloantibody to one or more of the hundreds of red blood cell antigens present. Any antigens that the patient does not possess are potentially immunogenic. Approximately 1.5-2.0% of hospital patients have detectable alloantibodies to red cell antigens caused by previous transfusion or pregnancy. The most frequently detected antibodies in order of decreasing frequency are; **D>K>E>CD>Fy^a>Jk^a>c >C>cE>e>DE>V>Jk^b**. Even components containing very few red blood cells, such as pooled random donor platelet concentrates can stimulate antibody formation.

Multiply transfused patients have much higher incidences of RBC antibody formation. The frequency varies with age and disease state. Overall, approximately 10% of patients transfused with multiple units of red blood cells form antibodies against some of the non-ABO, non-D antigens. In those patients who produce 1 RBC antibody, about 33% will produce additional antibodies.

Antibodies related to these antigens, like Rh antibodies, are unexpected and may interfere with compatibility testing. Some are immune, 37° reactive IgG antibodies and clinically significant because they are associated with transfusion reactions (TR) and HDN. Others are naturally occurring, cold reactive IgM antibodies and clinically insignificant because they are not usually associated with *in vivo* red cell destruction.

Clinical Significance of Most Common Blood Group Alloantibodies

Usually Clinically Significant	Sometimes Clinically Significant	Insignificant if not reactive at 37°C	Generally Clinically Insignificant
A&B	Colton	A$_1$	P^1
Diego	Dombrock	H	Sd^a
Duffy	Yt^a	M,N	Chido, Rodgers
Kell	Le^a		Cost
Kidd	Lutheran		Knops
Rh			Le^b
S,s,U			

Common blood group antibodies and their reactivity are summarized in the table on the next page.

Common Red Blood Cell Antibody Properties & Clinical Significance

Blood Group System	Antibody	Reactivity	TR	HDN	% Units Compatible	Transfuse
Rh	D	IAT	YES	YES	15	Antigen neg unit
	C	IAT	YES	YES	30	Antigen neg unit
	E	RT, IAT	YES	YES	70	Antigen neg unit
	c	IAT	YES	YES	20	Antigen neg unit
	e	IAT	YES	YES	3	Antigen neg unit
	C^w	RT, IAT	YES	YES	98	Antigen neg unit
Kell	K	RT, IAT	YES	YES	91	Antigen neg unit
	k	IAT	YES	YES	0.2	Antigen neg unit
	Kp^a	IAT	YES	YES	98	Antigen neg unit
	Kp^b	IAT	YES	YES	0	Antigen neg unit
	Js^a	IAT	YES	YES	100	Antigen neg unit
	Js^b	IAT	YES	YES	0	Antigen neg unit
Duffy	Fy^a	IAT	YES	YES	34	Antigen neg unit
	Fy^b	IAT	YES	YES	17	Antigen neg unit
Kidd	Jk^a	IAT	YES	YES	23	Antigen neg unit
	Jk^b	IAT	YES	YES	28	Antigen neg unit
Lewis	Le^a	RT, 37, IAT	RARE	NO	78	IAT XM compatible
	Le^b	RT, 37, IAT	NO	NO	22	IAT XM compatible
MNSs	M	RT, IAT	FEW	FEW	22	IAT XM compatible
	N	RT, IAT	NO	RARE	28	IAT XM compatible
	S	IAT	YES	YES	45	Ag neg unit
	s	IAT	YES	YES	11	Ag neg unit
P	P$_1$	RT	RARE	NO	21	IAT XM compatible
Lutheran	Lu^a	RT, IAT	NO	NO	92	IAT XM compatible
	Lu^b	RT, IAT	YES	YES	0.15	Medical decision

Abbreviations: IAT, indirect antiglobulin test; RT, room temperature; XM, crossmatch; neg, negative

- In the Kell blood group system, K is very immunogenic. K antigen occurs in only about 9% of Caucasians and 2% of African Americans.

- In the Duffy blood group system, the usual alleles are Fy^a and Fy^b. A third allele produces neither Fy^a nor Fy^b. Approximately 70% of African Americans lack both Fy^a and Fy^b.

- In the Kidd blood group system, about 77% of Caucasians express Jka (27% Jk^a Jk^a & 50% Jk^a Jk^b). The remaining 23% are Jk^b Jk^b. Most African Americans are Jk^a positive. Anti- Jk^a and Jk^b are IgG antibodies, but they invariably bind complement and may give stronger reactions in an indirect antiglobulin test with anti-C3 than with anti-IgG. In identifying anti-Jk^a a dosage effect is common, so that positive results may be obtained only with homozygous Jk^a Jk^a cells.

- Anti-Lewis a & b antibodies are usually IgM and are seldom clinically significant. They are commonly detected during pregnancy.

- In the MNSs system, anti-M and anti-N are usually IgM antibodies and are rarely clinically significant. Numerous low frequency antigens have been described in this system, but they have little practical significance. Anti-S antibodies are often IgG and reactive at 37o C.

- Almost all individuals are either P_1 (75%) or P_2. P_2 persons frequently have anti-P_1, which is usually an IgM antibody. Some anti-P antibodies behave as agglutinins at room temperature and as hemolysins at 37°C, which is termed biphasic hemolysis or Donath-Landsteiner antibodies. Anti-P autoantibody is associated with paroxysmal cold hemoglobinuria (PCH). Rare individuals with the p phenotype, who lack P_1, P and P^k antigens, make an antibody against all three antigens, termed anti-Tja (anti-P_1+P+P^k).

- About 8% of Caucasians are Lu^a positive; almost all of them are LuaLub. The remaining 92% of the population are $Lu^b Lu^b$. Anti-Lu^a is not associated with increased red cell destruction. Anti-Lub is rarely a cause of a delayed hemolytic transfusion reaction, but not HDN.

- Anti I is frequently associated with cold autoimmune hemolytic anemia (AIHA).

All detected antibodies are investigated and clinically significant ones are identified so that antigen negative blood can be provided for transfusion. If a patient has multiple antibodies, the percent of red cell units that will be compatible can be calculated in the following manner.

1. Find % units compatible for each antibody in table above.
2. Convert %compatible number to a decimal.
3. Multiply the decimal fraction of the 1st antibody by 2nd antibody and the 3rd antibody, etc.
4. Multiply the result by 100 and round off the result to the nearest whole number.
5. The answer is the percent of red cell units that will be compatible.

Example: A patient has anti-K (91% compatible), anti-E (70% compatible) and anti-Fy^a (34% compatible). The % units compatible = 0.91 x 0.70 x 0.34 = 0.22 x 100 = 22%

CONSEQUENCES OF RED BLOOD CELL ANTIBODIES

Some antibodies, particularly IgM antibodies of the ABO blood group system, are capable of fixing complement to the red cell surface. Complement is a plasma protein cascade that is activated by some antigen-antibody reactions. Binding of the membrane attack complex disrupts the cell membrane, causing hemolysis. Hemoglobin is released into the plasma, resulting in hemoglobinemia and hemoglobinuria. This process is termed intravascular hemolysis.

Red cells coated with IgG antibody that does not fix complement are removed from the circulation following phagocytosis by reticuloendothelial cells. During phagocytosis, heme is metabolized to bilirubin, resulting in icterus. Hemoglobinemia and hemoglobinuria do not occur. This process is termed extravascular hemolysis.

CHAPTER 2:
Compatibility Testing

Compatibility tests are performed in order to help prevent hemolytic transfusion reactions which may be caused by antibodies of the ABO blood group system or by antibodies to other blood group antigens.

Compatibility testing includes verification of the ABO & Rh type of the donor blood and the following tests on recipient's blood:

- ABO and Rh typing
- Antibody screen for unexpected antibodies
- Crossmatch between donor red cells and recipient serum.

TIMING OF COMPATIBILITY TESTING

A sample must be obtained from the patient within 3 days of the scheduled transfusion for compatibility testing if any of the following conditions exist:

- Patient has been transfused with a blood component containing red blood cells in the preceding 3 months
- Patient has been pregnant within the preceding 3 months
- Patient history is uncertain.

Testing of a new sample is necessary because a patient can develop a primary antibody response at any time within the first three months following immunization.

ABO TYPING

ABO typing is accomplished by:

- Testing patient's red cells with anti-A and anti-B antisera (forward typing)
- Testing patient's serum for anti-A and anti-B (back or reverse typing).

The ABO system is unique because plasma has naturally occurring antibodies to the ABO red cell antigens that are absent from his or her own red cells. These antibodies are the basis for ABO compatibility criteria when selecting red cells and plasma for transfusion.

Interpretation of ABO Typing

RBC + Anti-A	RBC + Anti-B	Serum + A cells	Serum + B cells	ABO Group	Compatible RBCs	Compatible Plasma
+	-	-	+	A	A, O	A, AB
-	+	+	-	B	B, O	B, AB
+	+	-	-	AB	AB, A, B, O	Only AB
-	-	+	+	O	Only O	O, A, B, AB

Determination of ABO blood groups is the most important pretransfusion compatibility test. If tests are done to insure that donor and recipient belong to the same ABO blood group, then even if no other tests are done, the donor's red blood cells will be compatible with the recipient's plasma in about 97% of cases.

Selection of RBC Units When ABO Specific Blood is not available.

When ABO specific blood is not available, it is important to use RBCs that are still compatible with the recipient's serum; that is, crossmatch compatible. Donor RBCs must not contain A or B antigens that react with the anti-A or anti-B present in the recipient's serum. In this situation the large amount of anti-A or anti-B in the recipient's plasma would bind to transfused ABO incompatible RBCs and cause hemolysis. The reverse situation, in which the recipient's RBCs have an antigen that reacts with an antibody in the donor's plasma, is not as important. In this case, the small amount of antibody present in the 100 mL of plasma remaining in a RBC unit is rapidly diluted about 30 fold in the recipient's plasma before the antibody can injure enough RBCs to be clinically apparent. The following table summarizes the proper selection of RBCs for Rh positive recipients when ABO group specific blood is unavailable.

RBC Selection When Type-Specific Blood is Unavailable

Recipient ABO Group	1st Choice RBC Unit	2nd Choice RBC Unit	3rd Choice RBC Unit
O+	O+	O-	None
A+	A+	O+	O-
B+	B+	O+	O-
AB+	AB+	A+	B+
O-	O-	O+	None
A-	A-	O-	A+
B-	B-	O-	B+ or O+
AB-	AB-	A-	B-

RH TYPING

Rh typing is performed so that Rh positive red blood cells will not be given to an Rh negative recipient. This prevents Rh immunization in patients without pre-existing anti-D and prevents hemolytic transfusion reactions in patients who have already developed anti-D antibodies.

The presence or absence of the D antigen in the Rh blood group system defines whether a person is Rh-positive or Rh-negative. About 85% of the US population is Rh positive and 15% is Rh negative.

In contrast to the ABO system, patients with D-negative red cells will not make anti-D unless they have been immunized previously by exposure to Rh positive red cells via fetomaternal transfer during pregnancy or prior transfusion.

Rh-positive recipients can receive Rh positive or Rh negative RBCs, but Rh-negative recipients should only receive Rh-negative blood. For Rh negative recipients, the order of choices is the same as far as ABO groups are concerned.

- Rh negative patients can be given Rh positive blood in an emergent situation if they lack anti-D antibody.
- Rh positive blood should not be given to patients who have previously demonstrated anti-D antibody.
- Rh positive blood should also be avoided, if possible, when transfusing Rh negative women of childbearing potential or Rh negative women who have had multiple pregnancies.

Multiparous patients may no longer have detectable anti-D antibody, but transfusion may cause an anamnestic response and a delayed hemolytic reaction. Administration of Rh positive blood to an Rh negative female of childbearing potential could stimulate the synthesis of anti-D IgG and cause hemolytic disease of the newborn during a subsequent pregnancy.

PRINCIPLES OF SEROLOGIC TESTS FOR RED CELL ANTIBODY DETECTION

When antibodies react with red cells, agglutination may occur particularly if the antibody is of the IgM class. Many IgG antibodies react with their corresponding antigen on the red cell but do not cause agglutination. For this reason, the anti-human globulin test (Coombs Test) was developed. Antibodies against human IgG and complement can react with red cells that are coated with non-agglutinating antibodies and/or with complement components and cause visible agglutination. These products are called anti-human globulin (AHG) reagents.

The antiglobulin test is either direct (DAT) or indirect (IAT). Medical applications of the DAT and IAT are summarized in the following table.

Medical Applicants of the Direct & Indirect Antiglobulin Tests

Direct Antiglobulin Test	Indirect Antiglobulin Test
Hemolytic disease of the newborn	Detection of unexpected antibodies in plasma (Antibody screen)
Autoimmune hemolytic anemia	Compatibility testing
Drug induced red cell sensitization	Detection of some RBC antigens not demonstrable by other techniques
Hemolytic transfusion reactions	

The direct antiglobulin test (DAT) is performed to determine if a patient's red cells are coated *in vivo* with IgG or complement components. In the DAT, red cells are taken from the patient, washed to remove unbound IgG and then directly tested with antiglobulin reagent (anti-IgG and/or anti-complement). If antibody is coating the patient's red cells, they are agglutinated by antiglobulin. The DAT is extremely sensitive; it can detect as few as 100 IgG and 400 C3d molecules per red cell.

Approximately 1 in 9000 healthy persons has a positive direct antiglobulin test with no evidence of hemolysis. Some diseases may be associated with a positive DAT, even though the patient does not appear to be actively hemolyzing their red cells. Examples include chronic lymphocytic leukemia, multiple myeloma, systemic lupus erythematosis, infectious mononucleosis, mycoplasma infection, and AIDS. Different studies have reported that 0.3 to 1.5% of hospitalized patients have a positive DAT.

Autoimmune hemolytic anemia is classified as warm or cold autoantiobody types based on the temperatures at which the antibodies maximally react with red blood cells *in vitro*. Warm autoantibodies are more reactive at 37°C than at lower temperatures, whereas cold autoantibodies react optimally at 5°C and less strongly at higher temperatures.

Characteristic Serological Findings in Autoimmune Hemolytic Anemias

Type of AIHA	DAT Result	Antibody Screen	Antibody Specificity
Warm antibody	IgG, C3 or both	Positive in 55%	Nonspecific or Rh
Cold Agglutinin	C3 alone	Positive up to 30°C	Anti-I or i
Paroxysmal Cold Hemoglobinuria	C3 alone	Biphasic hemolysin	Anti-P

In warm autoimmune hemolytic anemia, RBCs may be coated with IgG, IgG and complement, or complement alone. IgG is found alone in about 60% of cases and in association with complement in about 30% of cases. In contrast, cold autoimmune hemolytic anemia is caused by complement-fixing IgM antibodies. In these cases, the direct antiglobulin test detects only complement.

The following table lists numerous drugs that have been associated with a positive DAT.

Acetaminophen	Fenoprofen	6-mercaptopurine	Sulbactam
Amoxicillin	Fludarabine	Methicillin	Sulindac
Amphotericin	Fluoroquinolones	Methotrexate	Sulfonamides
Ampicillin	Fluorouracil	Methyldopa	Sulfasalazide
Carbenicillin	Hydralazine	Metrizoate contrast	Tazobactam
Carbimazole	Hydrochlorothiazide	Nafcillin	Teicoplanin
Carboplatin	Ibuprofen	Norfloxacine	Temafloxacin
Cephalosporins	Insulin	Oxaliplatin	Teniposide
Chlordiazepoxide	Interferon	Penicillin G	Tetracycline
Chlorpromazine	Interleukin 2	Piperacillin	Ticarcillin
Chlorporpamide	Isoniazid	Probenacid	Tolbutamide
Cisplatin	Latamoxef	Quinidine	Tolmetin
Clavulante	Levodopa	Quinine	Triamterene
Declofenac	Levofloxacin	Ranitidine	Zomepirac
Diphenylhydantoin	Mefenamic acid	Rifampicin	Zosyn
Erythromycin	Mefloquine	Streptokinase	
Etodolac	Melphalan	Streptomycin	

Drug induced hemolytic anemia is very rare. The incidence has been estimated to be one case per 1 million individuals. The most common cause of drug induced hemolytic anemia is the 2nd and 3rd generation cephalosporins. Of these, cefotetan appears to be the worst offender. The purine analogue, fludarabine, is used to treat chronic lymphocytic leukemia and produces a positive DAT in almost 35% of cases.

A DAT should be performed whenever there is:

- A physician order
- Hemolytic transfusion reaction investigation
- Hemolytic disease of the newborn investigation
- An antibody panel has a positive auto control
- An unexpected positive antiglobulin crossmatch (on donor RBCs)

The strength of the direct antiglobulin test does not predict the biological activity of antibodies. For instance, some patients with a strongly positive direct antiglobulin test have little hemolysis, while other patients with weakly positive or negative direct antiglobulin test hemolyze extensively. Also, the strength of the direct antiglobulin test often does not change following treatment, even though the clinical condition greatly improves.

In the indirect antiglobulin test (IAT), patient serum is incubated with commercially available normal red cells to allow in vitro coating of red cells. After incubation, the red cells are washed to remove unbound immunoglobulin and tested with anti-IgG. If antibody is present in the patient's serum, red cells become coated with antibody and are agglutinated by the antiglobulin reagent. Thus, the IAT detects the presence of antibody in serum. The major applications of the IAT are discussed in the following sections.

ANTIBODY SCREEN

The antibody screen detects alloantibodies and autoantibodies in patient plasma, which have specificity for red blood cells. Red cell antibodies are detectable in up to 2.6% of the general population and more commonly in individuals who have been previously transfused. This test is performed by incubating patient plasma with two or three commercially available group O RBCs that have been extensively antigen typed. The FDA mandates that red cells for antibody detection possess the following antigens: C, D, E, c, e, M, N, S, s, P1, Lea, Leb, K, k, Fya, Fyb, Jka, and JKb. Although not required, it is generally agreed that homozygosity for C, D, E, c, e, Fya and Jka is also preferable. The test is performed under conditions that detect clinically significant antibodies reactive at 37°C and the antiglobulin phase. It is designed to detect most unexpected antibodies to common red cell antigens other than anti-A or B.

Screening cells cannot possibly be positive for all of the antigens that have a low frequency. Therefore, it is possible to get a falsely negative antibody screen. For example, if a patient has an antibody to Kp^a and the screening cells are negative for Kp^a antigen, the antibody will not be detected. Fortunately, the incidence of Kp^a antigen is about 1%, so the likelihood of selecting a unit for immediate spin crossmatch that would be Kp^a positive is very low. However, if a Kp^a positive unit was selected, an immediate spin crossmatch would not detect any incompatibility and an incompatible unit would be transfused.

Antibody binding to red blood cells can be enhanced by manipulation of environmental conditions or the red cell membrane. In general, physiological temperature and pH promote red blood cell antigen- antibody interactions. The negative charge of red cell membranes causes red cells to naturally repel each other. Enzyme modification of red blood cells reduces net surface charge and distance between cells, facilitating red cell agglutination by IgG molecules. The enzymes used in detection of blood group antibodies include ficin, papain, and bromelin.

Suspension of red blood cells in low ionic strength solutions (LISS) decreases the ionic strength of the reaction medium and increases the attraction between positively charged IgG molecules and negatively charged red blood cells. Most LISS reagents contain 0.2% NaCl. LISS increases the rate of antibody binding to red blood cells and allows shorter incubation times.

Polyethylene glycol (PEG) is a macromolecular additive within a LISS that brings antibody sensitized red blood cells closer together and promotes antibody cross-linking and enhancement of agglutination reactions. PEG is more effective than LISS alone in detecting weak antibodies.

CROSSMATCH TESTS

If the antibody screen is negative and blood bank records show no previous history of antibody, the next step is to do an immediate spin crossmatch. The immediate spin crossmatch is sufficient to detect ABO incompatibility. However, if the antibody screen is positive, antibody identification and selection of antigen negative units must be completed prior to performing an AHG crossmatch (see next section).

A crossmatch consists of testing patient serum against a sample of red cells from the actual unit that has been selected for transfusion. There are two types of crossmatches:

1. The immediate spin crossmatch is performed by mixing patient plasma with a sample of RBCs from the unit selected for transfusion and observing for immediate agglutination and/or hemolysis that is caused by ABO antibodies. An immediate spin crossmatch takes about 5 minutes to perform.

2. An AHG crossmatch (antiglobulin crossmatch) is performed by incubating patient plasma with a sample of red cells from the unit to be transfused in the presence of LISS or PEG. The tube is centrifuged and observed for agglutination prior to performing the antiglobulin test. An AHG crossmatch test takes about 30 minutes to complete.

Several studies have shown that there is a small risk of missing antibodies when the antiglobulin phase of the crossmatch is not performed. The risk has been estimated to be 1 miss per 10,000 crossmatches. However, the risk that one of these missed antibodies will cause a hemolytic transfusion reaction is only 1 case per 500,000 crossmatches.

Any blood component containing a significant number of RBCs needs to be crossmatched prior to transfusion including red blood cells, leukocyte reduced red blood cells, saline washed red blood cells, and granulocytes

The following information must be included with a crossmatch request:

1. Component desired.
2. Number of units needed.
3. Transfusion priority such as Hold, Give, Surgery.
4. Date of transfusion or surgery.

ANTIBODY SCREEN & AHG CROSSMATCH DISCREPANCIES

The antibody screen can sometimes be positive when one or more of the crossmatches are negative. Some reasons are:

*   Antibody screening red cells express antigens that crossmatched units do not. Common examples include moderate frequency antigens such as K, Lu^a, Co^b and Yt^b.
*   Antibody screening red cells express a double dose of an antigen (e.g. JK(a+b-), but crossmatched red cells express a single dose (e.g. Jk(a+b+).

Occasionally, one or more crossmatches may be positive when the antibody screen is negative. This discrepancy may occur because:

*   Antibody screening red cells are group O and the antibodies are anti-A or anti-B.
*   A low to moderate frequency antigen is present on the crossmatched red cells, but not on the antibody screening red cells. Examples include: Wr^a, Kp^a, Js^a, C^w, Di^a, Go^a, Sc2, Mi^a, Lu^a, Co^b and Yt^b.
*   Antibody screening red cells may not have antigens such as f (ce). For example, CDe and cDE antibody screening cells will not be f+, but cde crossmatched units may be f+.
*   Crossmatched red cells are usually fresher than antibody screening red cells. RBC antigens get weaker during storage and very weak antibodies may react more strongly with fresher red cells. Xga antigen seems to be especially prone to deteriorate during storage.
*   Crossmatched red cells may express a double dose of an antigen (e.g. Jk(a+b-)) and the antibody screening red cells a single dose (e.g. Jk(a+b+)).

ANTIBODY IDENTIFICATION

If the antibody screen is positive, the specificity of the antibody is identified by testing the serum against a panel of 8 to 20 Group O RBCs of varying phenotypes. The pattern of positive and negative reactions with these cells identifies the antigen against which the antibody is directed. Antibody identification is accomplished by the "crossing out" method which consists of identifying each cell that is negative and crossing out all of the antigens present on that cell. The panel should also be observed to:

- Determine if the antibody is stronger at room temperature, 37°C, or antiglobulin phase
- Determine if the auto control is negative or positive.

From this information, one can determine:

- Identity of the antibody
- If the antibody is an alloantibody or alloantibody
- If an autoantibody is cold or warm.

Antibody Panel Interpretation

Thermal Characteristic	Pattern of Reactivity	Auto Control	Interpretation
Stronger at cold & weaker at warm temperatures	One or few cells positive	Negative	Consider cold alloantibody such as MN, P, Le, etc.
Stronger at cold & weaker at warm temperatures	All cells positive	Negative	Consider Vel, Tj^a, etc
Stronger at cold & weaker at warm temperatures	All cells positive	Positive	Cold autoantibody such as anti-I
Negative in cold & positive at warmer temperatures	One or few cells positive	Negative	Consider clinically significant alloantibody such as Rh, Kell, Duffy, Kidd, Ss, etc.
Negative in cold & positive at warmer temperatures	All cells positive	Negative	Consider alloantibody to high frequency antigen, KP^b, k, Lu^b, Js^b, Lan, Ge, At^a, U, etc.
Negative in cold & positive at warmer temperatures	All cells positive	Positive	Consider autoantibody with or without alloantibody

If a clinically significant antibody is identified, only red cells negative for the relevant antigen will be selected for crossmatching and transfusion. For example, if the antibody is anti-K, RBC of the appropriate ABO and Rh type will be tested with anti-K anti-serum and only K-negative red cells will be selected for transfusion. For added safety, an AHG crossmatch is also performed. For clinically insignificant antibodies, it is permissible to crossmatch units that have not been antigen typed.

When the antibody screen is positive, additional time is required to identify the antibody(ies), to find antigen-negative red cells, and to perform AHG crossmatches. This time can range from an hour to days if multiple antibodies, antibodies against high frequency antigens, or a mixture of autoantibody and alloantibodies are present. If transfusion is medically necessary before compatible blood can be obtained, the attending physician and the transfusion medicine physician need to discuss the risk : benefit ratio of transfusing potentially incompatible blood.

Autoantibodies

An autoantibody is produced against a person's own red cells. When a patient has an autoantibody, the direct antiglobulin test and the auto control in an antibody panel will be positive. In addition, all cells in the panel will be reactive. If the antibody reactions are stronger at colder temperatures and weaker at warm temperatures, the patient probably has a cold autoantibody. If the antibody reactions are negative at colder temperatures and positive at warmer temperatures, the patient most likely has a warm autoantibody.

ADSORPTION PROCEDURES

Sometimes, patients with autoantibodies require red cell transfusion. The most important technical issue faced by the transfusion service is determining if the patient's serum contains alloantibodies in addition to the autoantibody. Between 15 and 40% of patients with autoimmune hemolytic anemia have alloantibodies. The most common alloantibodies detected in the sera of patients with AIHA in descending order are: anti-E, K, C, Fy^a, Jk^a, and c.

The most frequently used method for detecting alloantibodies in the presence of a broadly reactive autoantibody is the warm auto adsorption procedure. Autoantibody is removed from autologous red cells by heat or chemical treatment and then the red cells are treated with an enzyme to enhance autoantibody adsorption. The most popular technique is to treat red cells with ZZAP, which is a combination of dithiothreitol and papain. Autoantibody is then absorbed from plasma with these treated autologous red cells. Several adsorptions may be necessary to remove all of the autoantibody. If no antibody is detected, the adsorbed plasma can be used for crossmatching donor units. If alloantibody is present, it must be identified and antigen negative units selected for crossmatching.

The warm auto adsorption procedure is not useful in patients who have been transfused within the past 30 days because even a small percentage of transfused cells may adsorb alloantibody, producing a falsely negative result. In this situation, allogeneic adsorptions may be required. By selecting two or three samples of red cells of varying phenotypes, almost all clinically significant alloantibodies can be detected. For example, adsorbing a serum containing an autoantibody and an anti-Jk^a alloantibody with Jk^a negative red cells will remove the autoantibody but not the anti-Jk^a. Once the autoantibody is removed, the remaining alloantibodies can be identified using a panel. This procedure is usually performed at a blood center reference laboratory instead of a hospital transfusion service.

Compatibility Testing Overview

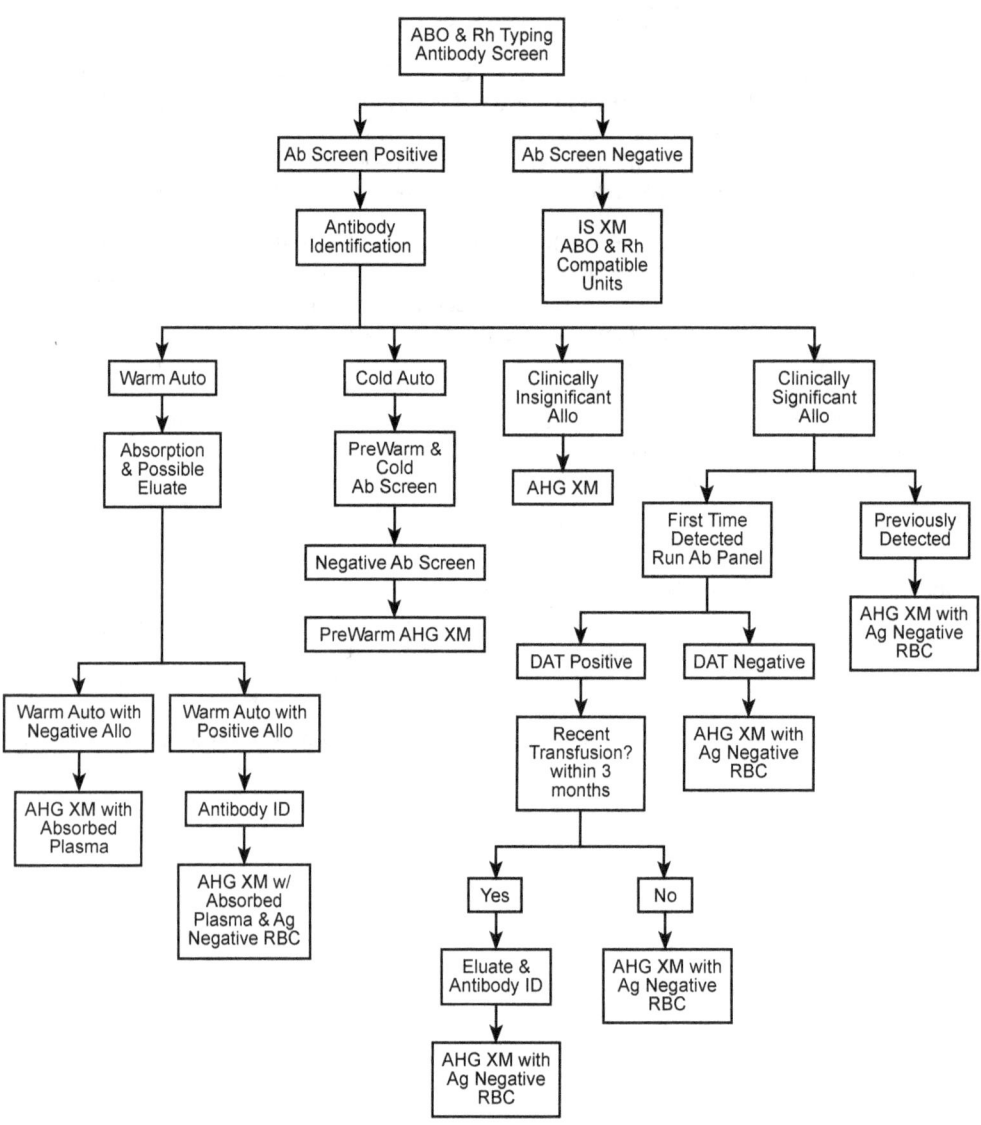

ORDERING BLOOD FOR SURGERY

Type and Crossmatch
If it is likely that a patient will require transfusion, then the physician should order a type and crossmatch of an appropriate number of units. This order will insure that blood will be available at the time of surgery. Blood crossmatched for surgery and not transfused is usually released the morning after surgery.

Type and Screen
A type and screen should be ordered when there is a reasonable possibility that a surgical patient will require blood but the likelihood of transfusion is too low to justify reserving crossmatched units. As a general guideline, if a surgical procedure requires transfusion in less than 10% of cases, a type and screen rather than type and crossmatch is appropriate.

When a type and screen is ordered, ABO and Rh typing and antibody screen are performed. This allows the Transfusion Service to identify patients with unusual blood types or complex antibodies ahead of time so that problems can be resolved prior to surgery.

If a patient requires blood during surgery, and the antibody screen is negative, units are issued after an immediate spin crossmatch. This process takes 5 to 10 minutes. If clinically significant antibodies are detected during the antibody screen, antigen-negative units are identified and crossmatched using AHG.

Maximum Surgical Blood Order Schedule
A Maximum Surgical Blood Order Schedule (MSBOS) is a listing of surgical procedures performed at a given institution with recommended maximum blood orders for each procedure These blood orders are based on actual intraoperative blood use at the institution and are typically set to cover 90% of patient needs. MSBOS is a useful guideline for surgical blood ordering. Blood orders may be periodically monitored by the blood bank staff to assure conformity with these guidelines.

Emergency Transfusion
In an emergency, the patient's physician must weigh the risk of transfusing uncrossmatched blood against the hazard of waiting for a completed crossmatch. If the physician believes the urgency of the situation warrants the use of uncrossmatched blood, they are aksed to sign an Emergency Blood Release Form to document the reason for the urgent need and to acknowledge that units are not crossmatched at the time of transfusion. Direct consultation with Blood Bank personnel is highly recommended to expedite requests. Two options are available for emergency transfusion. O-negative red cells are available for immediate transfusion to any patient, but should be used only when the patient's blood type is not known and there is insufficient time for typing. This situation will sometimes occur in the trauma setting and should only apply to the first few units given. The preferred medical practice is to transfuse ABO type-specific blood rather than O-negative red cells whenever possible in order to conserve the O-negative blood supply and to minimize transfusion of potentially incompatible group O plasma. Blood typing can be completed and type-specific blood made available within 5 minutes after receipt of a patient sample. Blood type cards or dog tags from other facilities are not acceptable documentation of blood type.

In all emergency situations, standard compatibility testing for units issued uncrossmatched is initiated and completed without delay and additional crossmatched blood is made available as soon as possible. If any compatibility problem is detected during follow-up testing, the physician is notified immediately.

CIRCUMSTANCES IN WHICH IT IS DIFFICULT OR IMPOSSIBLE TO FIND COMPATIBLE BLOOD

Some patients have multiple red cell alloantibodies. For example, when a patient has anti-Fya, anti-Jkb, anti-E and anti-S, blood bank technologists will test units of the appropriate ABO type until they find units that are negative for all four antigens and then must perform an AHG crossmatch. In the example given, the probability of a given unit of red cells lacking all four antigens is 3% (1 in 33 units). If transfusion is required on an emergency basis or if large numbers of units are required urgently, it may be impossible to supply antigen-negative blood.

Patients with alloantibody to an antigen that is on an extremely high percentage of homologous red cells (i.e., a high frequency antigen) may be incompatible with all red cells tested. Some of these antibodies are clinically insignificant but others may cause shortened red cell survival. In these cases, the regional blood center may have to search for suitable donors among family members or rare donor files.

Some patients have red cell autoantibodies that react with all homologous red cells tested. In this instance, it is almost impossible to provide compatible blood for transfusion. For extreme life-threatening emergencies, utilization of blood that one expects may be hemolyzed rapidly is nevertheless warranted, particularly since such dire expectations are not always realized.

In Vivo Compatibility Test

The presence of an antibody in a patient's plasma does not necessarily indicate that transfusion of incompatible blood will result in shortened survival of transfused red cells. When no compatible red blood cells can be found by *in vitro* compatibility testing and the need for transfusion is urgent, then an *in vivo* crossmatch might be helpful in assessing the possible outcome of a transfusion. The principle underlying this test is that intravascular hemolysis of as little as 5 mL of red cells will raise the plasma hemoglobin concentration of an adult by about 50 mg/dL, which is an amount that can be easily visualized.

The medical director of the hospital transfusion service in consultation with the patient's physician must approve an in vivo crossmatch before it is undertaken. The most practical method is to:

- Infuse an aliquot of 25 to 50 mL of Red Blood Cells from the unit to be transfused over a period of 20 to 30 minutes.
- Carefully observe the patient for symptoms of a hemolytic transfusion reaction throughout the infusion.
- Discontinue the infusion and keep the line open with saline.
- Draw 5 mL of blood into a lavender (EDTA) vacutainer tube.
- Centrifuge the tube to separate the cells from the plasma.
- Observe the plasma for hemolysis.
- If no hemolysis is observed, the remainder of the unit may be transfused cautiously.

Lack of hemoglobinemia suggests that immediate catastrophic hemolysis will not occur with infusion of the entire unit of blood, but does not guarantee that the infusion of the remainder of the unit will not cause an adverse reaction. If a patient tolerates 3 units of Red Blood Cells with no reactions, the in vivo crossmatch may be discontinued after the 3rd unit.

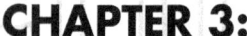

CHAPTER 3:
Prenatal and Perinatal Immunohematologic Testing

There are three main objectives of prenatal and perinatal testing:

- Identify Rh negative women
- Identify women with clinically significant alloantibodies
- Assist in the diagnosis and management of hemolytic disease of the newborn

PRENATAL TESTING

Current recommendations for prenatal testing are summarized in the following table.

Prenatal Testing Guidelines

Test	Situation	Timing
ABO Typing	Pregnancy	Initial visit
Rh Typing	Pregnancy	Initial visit & 26-29 weeks
Antibody Screen	All Pregnancies	Initial visit
	D negative pregnancy	Before RhIg therapy
	D positive pregnancy	3rd trimester if history of antibodies or transfusion
Antibody ID	Positive antibody screen	Upon detection
Antibody titer	Rh or other clinically significant antibody	Upon initial detection
		Repeat at 18-20 weeks
		Repeat at 2-4 week intervals if below critical titer

All women should be tested for ABO and D as early as possible in pregnancy, preferably during their first trimester visit. ABO typing is done primarily for patient identification. The results should not conflict with historical records. Any discrepant results must be fully investigated. A record of the maternal ABO type is also helpful should the newborn infant develop signs and symptoms consistent with ABO HDN.

D typing should be done on at least two separate occasions and the results should be identical. This recommendation is especially important as a safeguard to prevent an Rh negative woman from being falsely typed as Rh positive and denied RhIG. Serologic confirmation of the D type is also recommended at the beginning of each subsequent pregnancy.

Historically, if a patient typed as Rh negative, additional testing was then performed to determine if they had weak D expression. The AABB has determined that weak D testing is no longer necessary for obstetric patients. The main reason is that today's blood typing reagents are much more potent and most of the patients who were previously typed as weak D are now typed as Rh positive. All women are now typed as either Rh negative or positive. The clinical implication of this change is that a few women who actually have weak expression of the D antigen will be classified as Rh negative and will be candidates for Rh immune globulin. Giving Rh immune globulin to these women is not harmful.

All women, regardless of their D type, should be tested during each pregnancy for clinically significant antibodies, ideally at their first obstetrician visit. Antiglobulin testing should be done with anti-IgG reagent to detect clinically significant antibodies that are capable of crossing the placenta and causing hemolytic disease of the newborn (HDN). The same enhancement methods (LISS, PEG) used to detect unexpected antibodies during pretransfusion testing can be used for prenatal antibody detection.

An additional antibody screen may be ordered for Rh negative women at 26 to 28 weeks gestation to determine if active immunity to D has developed, before administration of RhIG prophylaxis. The risk of a woman developing anti-D between the first trimester and 28 weeks gestation is very low, occurring in only 2 of every 1000 Rh negative pregnancies. This antibody screen is not required by regulatory agencies and is probably not cost effective.

In most cases, Rh positive patients need be screened for antibodies only once during their initial visit. Only 1 in every 1000 women develops new antibodies capable of causing HDN between the first and third trimesters. Routine testing for unexpected antibodies in the third trimester or at delivery rarely provides useful clinical information.

Regardless of D type, additional antibody screening in the third trimester is indicated when there is a history of significant antibodies, blood transfusions or traumatic deliveries. Antibody screening is also necessary prior to antepartum transfusion.

If the antibody screen is positive at any time during pregnancy, the blood group specificity of the antibody should be identified. It should not be assumed that an antibody present in a D negative woman is anti-D, even after RhIG therapy. A limited panel or Rh negative RBCs, consisting of r'r (dCe/dce), r''r (dcE/dce), and rr (dce/dce) cells, can be used to exclude significant antibodies other than D. If the results of this limited panel are negative, it can be concluded that the original antibody screen was positive due to anti-D.

If a pregnant woman's plasma is reactive with one or more of the limited panel cells, then a comprehensive antibody panel needs to be run to identify antibody specificity. Antibody identification is necessary to determine if the antibody is likely to cause HDN (refer to table in Chapter 1). IgG antibodies to Rh, Kell, Duffy, Kidd and S antigens are likely to cause HDN. Some IgG antibodies, such as antibodies to Chido/Rodgers, Knops and Cromer system antigens, usually do not cause HDN. Antibodies to Lewis, P1 and M antigens are usually IgM and do not cross the placenta. Also, these antigens are poorly expressed on fetal RBCs. Even if antibody did cross the placenta, it would not bind to fetal RBCs. Therefore, HDN is unlikely. Once these IgM antibodies are identified, no further testing is required.

Once a clinically significant antibody is identified, the titer needs to be measured to assist the obstetrician in determining the severity of HDN. In the first pregnancy affected with anti-D, either a rising titer or a critical titer of 16 indicates the need for close clinical monitoring. The critical titer varies from institution to institution, depending on the titer method, but is usually between 8 and 32. For anti-D, the use of R^2R^2 RBCs are recommended for titrations, because they have a uniform expression of D antigen from one donor to another. The introduction of Doppler ultrasonography of fetal cerebral blood flow has allowed for noninvasive assessment of fetal anemia due to immune hemolysis. Amniocentesis for OD450 determination is seldom necessary.

Transfusion services usually use the same critical titer as anti-D for other Rh antibodies. Very little data exists concerning critical titers for non-Rh antibodies encountered in pregnancy. Transfusion services may use a higher titer of 32 or 64 for these antibodies.

Repeat titers at 2 to 4 week intervals after 18 weeks gestation is helpful in determining the need for invasive monitoring. If a previous sample from the current pregnancy is available, it should be tested in parallel with the current sample. Once the decision has been made to monitor HDN with an invasive procedure, subsequent antibody titrations are not necessary.

Not all clinically significant antibodies detected during pregnancy will cause HDN. The mother's antibody may have been induced during a previous pregnancy by a different consort, in which case the current fetus may be antigen negative and not at risk for HDN. It is worthwhile to phenotype RBCs from the putative father whenever the potential for HDN exists. The probability that a fetus carries the antigen to which the maternal serum contains antibody can be estimated from maternal and paternal phenotypes. If there is a high likelihood that the father is heterozygous for the gene encoding the offending antigen, molecular genotyping of amniotic fluid cells or chorionic villi can be performed. Molecular assays are available for Rh, Kell, Duffy or Kidd genotypes.

TESTING AT DELIVERY

At delivery, the following tests should be performed on the mother.

- ABO and D typing should be performed if there is no record of two concordant results.
- ABO and D typing and antibody screening should be done if a type and crossmatch is ordered for transfusion.
- A test for fetal maternal hemorrhage (FMH) should be performed approximately one hour after delivery on a maternal sample from all Rh negative women who deliver a Rh positive fetus.

Testing for FMH should be done regardless of the presence of detectable passive anti-D in maternal serum. The rosette test is a useful screening method for FMH. A suspension of maternal blood is incubated with anti-D. The anti-D will bind to any Rh positive fetal RBCs present in the suspension. Indicator Rh positive cells are then added, which bind to anti-D coated fetal Rh positive cells, forming visible agglutinates (rosettes) around them. A fetal bleed of as little as 2.5 mL of fetal blood can be detected with this method. If the rosette test is positive, the degree of FMH can be quantified by using the Kleihauer Betke acid elution method or flow cytometry. The rosette test will not detect fetal RBCs with a weak D phenotype.

The Kleihauer Betke test relies on the principle that red cells containing fetal hemoglobin (HbF) are less susceptible to acid elution than cells containing HbA. A thin smear of maternal blood is exposed to citric acid, which elutes hemoglobin from maternal red cells, resulting in pale ghost cells. Fetal red cells are resistant to acid and retain their hemoglobin. Consequently, they stain pink with erythrosin B dye. The smear is examined microscopically to determine the percentage of fetal red blood cells. Results are reported as the percent of fetal RBCs seen. The sensitivity of the method is approximately 0.1 mL of fetal blood in the maternal circulation. This corresponds to about 1 fetal cell per 50,000 maternal cells. The Kleihauer-Betke stain may occasionally underestimate the number of fetal RBCs present due to the fact that the fetus begins to synthesize hemoglobin A in the last trimester of pregnancy. Fetal cells, which had completed the switch to adult hemoglobin, would be counted as adult cells. False positive reactions may occur when maternal RBCs have increased levels of hemoglobin F such as occurs in various hemoglobinopathies including hereditary persistence of fetal hemoglobin, thalassemias, and sickle cell anemia.

This test involves a considerable amount of subjective interpretation. The quality of the stain must be very good so that red cells can be clearly distinguished from leukocytes. Several published studies and proficiency surveys have demonstrated that the precision and accuracy of this method are poor. Variation from laboratory to laboratory is 50% and the rate of fetal cell detection is only 90%.

The flow cytometric method utilizes a fluorescently labeled monoclonal antibody to the gamma chain of the HbF molecule (anti-HbF). A sample of whole blood is fixed with glutaraldehyde to crosslink hemoglobin inside the cells and then cell membranes are permeabilized with a detergent to ensure access and binding of anti-HbF. A flow cytometer determines the percentage of fetal cells by analyzing approximately 65,000 cells. Fetal red cells are clearly distinguished from adult cells by their significantly higher fluorescent signal. Proficiency surveys have shown this method to be more accurate and precise. The coefficient of variation is <7.5%.

After delivery the following tests should be performed on a cord or newborn infant capillary or venous blood sample.

- ABO and Rh typing and a direct antiglobulin test are performed on infants born to group O women. This practice helps to identify those infants at risk of ABO HDN.

- ABO and Rh typing and a direct antiglobulin test should be performed on an infant if the mother was not tested for ABO, Rh and unexpected antibodies during pregnancy.

- Blood from infants born to Rh negative women should be tested for ABO and D, including weak D. If the infant has a weak D phenotype, the mother is a candidate for RhIG.

In the absence of maternal alloimmunization during pregnancy, serological testing of infant blood may be necessary if the baby develops unexplained jaundice or anemia. Initial tests should focus on detecting ABO incompatibility between fetus and mother. An ABO and Rh type and direct antiglobulin test should be performed, even though the DAT is often negative in ABO HDN. When ABO incompatibility exists, infant's plasma can be tested for unexpected antibodies against reagent group O, group A1 and/or group B RBCs. The presence of maternally derived IgG anti-A or anti-B in infant's plasma is sufficient evidence to support a diagnosis of ABO HDN.

CHAPTER 4:
Blood Donation

There are 3 categories of blood donors:

- Autologous donors give blood for their own use only, usually prior to a scheduled surgery.
- Allogenic or homologous donors give blood for someone else's use.
- Directed donors are a subcategory of allogeneic donors who donate for a designated patient.

ALLOGENEIC DONATIONS

General Donor Requirements
Allogenic blood donors should be 17 years or older, weigh 110 pounds or more, and should not have donated blood in the past 8 weeks. They must be in good health and feel well on the day of donation. They must have a negative history for hepatitis or jaundice after the age of 11 and not participate in any high risk behavior associated with HIV transmission. They should also be free of cancer and heart disease.

Donation Process
The total donation process takes about 1 hour and includes taking a medical history, donating blood and an observational recovery period. The blood collection facility has the responsibility of protecting both the donor and the recipient. The donor must answer very specific questions about his/her health and high risk activity practices. These questions are designed to prevent injury to the donor during donation and to prevent transmission of an infectious or other harmful agent to the recipient. The questions contained in the Uniform Donor History Questionnaire include:

Are you

1. Feeling healthy and well today?
2. Currently taking an antibiotic?
3. Currently taking any other medication for an infection?
4. Are you now taking or have you ever taken any medications on the Medication Deferral List (Proscar, Propecia, Avodart, Accutane, Soriatane, Tegison, growth hormone from human pituitary glands, bovine insulin, hepatitis B immune globulin, or unlicensed vaccine)?
5. Have you read the educational materials and had your questions answered?

In the past **48 hours**

6. Have you taken aspirin or anything that has aspirin in it?

In the past **6 weeks**

7. Female donors: Have you been pregnant or are you pregnant now?

In the past **8 weeks have you**

8. Donated blood, platelets or plasma?
9. Had any vaccinations or other shots?
10. Had contact with someone who had a smallpox vaccination?

In the past **16 weeks**

11. Have you donated a double unit of red cells using an apheresis machine?

In the past **12 months have you**

12. Had a blood transfusion?
13. Had a transplant such as organ, tissue, or bone marrow?
14. Had a graft such as bone or skin?
15. Come into contact with someone else's blood?
16. Had an accidental needle-stick?
17. Had sexual contact with anyone who has HIV/AIDS or has had a positive test for the HIV/AIDS virus?
18. Had sexual contact with a prostitute or anyone else who takes money or drugs or other payment for sex?
19. Had sexual contact with anyone who has ever used needles to take drugs or steroids, or anything not prescribed by their doctor?
20. Had sexual contact with anyone who has hemophilia or has used clotting factor concentrates?
21. Female donors: Had sexual contact with a male who has ever had sexual contact with another male?
22. Had sexual contact with a person who has hepatitis?
23. Lived with a person who has hepatitis?
24. Had a tattoo?
25. Had ear or body piercing?
26. Had or been treated for syphilis or gonorrhea?
27. Been in juvenile detention, lockup, jail, or prison for more than 72 hours?

In the past **three years have you**

28. Been outside the United States or Canada?

From **1980 through 1996,**

29. Did you spend time that adds up to three (3) months or more in the United Kingdom?
30. Were you a member of the U.S. military, a civilian military employee, or a dependent of a member of the U.S. military?

From **1980 to the present, did you**

31. Spend time that adds up to five (5) years or more in Europe?
32. Receive a blood transfusion in the United Kingdom?

From **1977 to the present, have you**

33. Received money, drugs, or other payment for sex?
34. Male donors: had sexual contact with another male, even once?

Have you **EVER**

35. Had a positive test for the HIV/AIDS virus?
36. Used needles to take drugs, steroids, or anything not prescribed by your doctor?
37. Used clotting factor concentrates?
38. Had hepatitis?
39. Had malaria?

40. Had Chagas' disease?

41. Had babesiosis?

42. Received a dura mater (or brain covering) graft?

43. Had any type of cancer, including leukemia?

44. Had any problems with your heart or lungs?

45. Had a bleeding condition or a blood disease?

46. Had sexual contact with anyone who was born in or lived in Africa?

47. Been in Africa?

48. Have any of your relatives had Creutzfeldt-Jakob disease?

Physical Exam

During the medical review a physical exam is performed to document weight, temperature, pulse, blood pressure, hemoglobin or hematocrit. The donor's arm is inspected to look for skin lesions and signs of possible IV drug abuse.

General Allogeneic Donor Physical Exam Criteria

Physical Attribute	Criteria
Age	At least 16 years old
Temperature	<37.5°C
Hemoglobin-Hematocrit	12.5 mg/dL (38% Hct)
Blood pressure	<180/100
Pulse	>50 and regular
Weight	Minimum of 110 lbs
Minimum Donation Interval	8 weeks (exceptions can be made)

Donor Deferral Rate

Approximately 15% of blood donors are deferred prior to donation because they do not meet one or more of the medical history or physical exam criteria. Low hemoglobin accounts for almost half of all deferrals.

Blood Donation

Blood is collected using aseptic technique and a sterile, FDA-approved collection bag. Equipment comes as single-use, disposable items, so donors cannot contract hepatitis or AIDS during blood donation. Approximately 450 mL of whole blood is collected into the blood bag. An additional 20-30 mL blood is collected into tubes for laboratory testing. The total amount withdrawn is 10 to 12% of the donor's total blood volume.

Only 1 to 2% of donors experience an adverse reaction to the donation. The most common problem is a vasovagal reaction. Symptoms may include transient low blood pressure, light-headedness, or fainting during or following the donation. Symptoms usually resolve within minutes.

Recovery Period

After donation, donors are required to rest for 15 minutes and take some refreshments. Post phlebotomy instructions recommend drinking more fluids than usual and avoiding immediate use of cigarettes or alcohol. Most donors resume normal activity after 30 minutes. However, donors with high risk occupations or hobbies (policemen, construction workers, pilots, etc) should consider special precautions. With adequate fluid intake, blood volume is restored within 12 hours, but red cell volume is not restored for several weeks.

Donor Testing

The tubes of blood collected with the donor unit are used for testing in accordance with American Association of Blood Banks (AABB) and federal regulations. These are described in the FDA required Circular of Information for the Use of Human Blood and Blood Components and are summarized below.

ABO & Rh type - Results are indicated in large letters on the label.

Antibody Screen - Only donors with a history of transfusion or pregnancy need be tested for unexpected red cell antibodies. However, most collecting facilities perform this test on all donors. When such antibodies are found the plasma portion of the unit is not used for allogenic transfusion.

Infectious Disease Tests - An increasing number of serologic and nucleic acid amplification tests have been added since the 1970's to detect infectious diseases.

Chronology of Blood Donor Testing

Year	Test
1972	Label blood from paid donors
1975	3rd generation test for HBsAg
1983	Exclusion of donors with high risk activities
1985	HIV antibody test
1987	ALT as surrogate test for HCV
1988	Anti-HBc as surrogate test for HCV
1989	HTLV-1 antibody test
1990	HCV antibody test
1992	2nd generation HCV antibody test
1993	HIV - 1 & 2 antibody test
1994	HTLV 1 & 2 antibody test
1995	HIV p24 antigen test
1999	NAT testing for HIV-1 & HCV
2003	NAT testing for West Nile Virus
2004	Bacterial culture of apheresis platelets
2007	Trypanosoma cruzi antibody

The infectious disease tests performed at each donation are summarized below.

Serologic Test for Syphilis – This test was initiated in the 1940's. It is known that acquiring syphilis from a transfusion is extremely rare. The risk appears more theoretical than real because donors with a history of gonorrhea or syphilis in the past 12 months are deferred and treponemes do not survivev more than 72 hours in refrigerated blood. Although its use is justified as an indicator for high risk behavior there are no data to support this assumption.

Hepatitis B Surface Antigen (HBsAg) – A radioimmunoassay was introduced in the early 1970s to detect hepatitis B virus carriers and was later replaced with an enzyme immunoassay (EIA).

Antibody to Human Immunodeficiency Virus (Anti-HIV) – An EIA was licensed by the FDA in March 1985. Reactive screening tests are confirmed with either Western Blot or immunofluorescence testing. Current methods detect infection with either HIV-1 or HIV-2.

Antibody to Hepatitis B Core Antigen (Anti-HBc) – An EIA was initiated in November 1986 as an indirect or surrogate marker for non-A,non-B hepatitis. The test was licensed by the FDA in 1990 as a test to further reduce the transmission of Hepatitis B. This test has many false positives and has poor specificity.

Alanine Aminotransferase (ALT) – Measurement of serum enzyme activity was introduced in November 1986 as a surrogate marker for non-A,non-B hepatitis. ALT has very poor specificity for viral hepatitis. ALT levels have not been required for volunteer blood donors in the U.S. since July 1995, but are still performed due to requirements for source plasma.

Antibody to Human T-cell Lymphotrophic Virus I & II (Anti-HTLV 1/II) – An EIA was implemented in February 1989. Current kits detect both HTLV-I and HTLV-II. A complicated algorithm is followed to distinguish between these two viruses that involves a second manufacturer's EIA, immunofluorescent antibody test, and recombinant immunoprecipitation assay (RIPA).

Antibody to Hepatitis C Virus (Anti-HCV) – An EIA was implemented in May, 1990 to detect donors exposed to HCV, previously called non-A, non-B hepatitis. A second generation test was introduced in 1992 and a third generation test in 1994.

HIV-1 p24 Antigen – An EIA was licensed in March 1996 as an additional test to prevent HIV transmission from donors who are in the early stages of infection and who have not yet developed antibody. The addition of HIV antigen testing reduced the window period between the time that a person contracts HIV and when the viruses can be detected from 22 days with HIV antibody alone to 16 days. FDA allowed HIV antigen testing to be discontinued after licensing of the NAT HIV test.

NAT for HCV & HIV – Nucleic Acid Testing for HCV & HIV was introduced to test minipools of plasma from 16 donors as a clinical trial under an investigational new drug (IND) protocol in June 1999. FDA licensed the first nucleic acid test system for the simultaneous detection of HIV and HCV RNA on Feb. 28, 2002. NAT has reduced the window period for HCV from 70 days (with EIA) to 10 days and for HIV from 22 days to 11 days. Approximately 4 per 1 million blood donations are from donors who are anti-HCV negative and HCV RNA positive.

NAT for West Nile Virus: Nucleic acid testing for West Nile Virus was introduced July 2003. Originally donor samples were tested in mini-pools. In 2008, AABB recommended that blood centers convert to individual testing whenever 2 presumed viremic donations are detected within a rolling seven day period. Facilities in geographic areas with ongoing WNV activity were advised to consider continuing individual testing for 14 days. Facilities can revert back to mini-pool testing after a minimum of 7 days without a presumed positive donation.

Bacterial culture: A method to limit or detect bacteria in all platelet products was implemented in 2004. Each apheresis platelet unit is cultured from the first day after collection until it outdates. If bacterial growth is detected in a unit, a blood center immediately notifies the hospital transfusion service.

Antibody toTrypanosoma cruzi:
Antibody testing for T. cruzi was introduced in 2007. FDA requires hospitals to participate in a Look-back program which involves identification of all recipients of previously transfused blood components from confirmed positive donors.

Donations with reactive test results are destroyed regardless of subsequently obtained confirmatory test results as a precautionary measure to prevent infectious units from entering the blood supply. Donors with abnormal tests are notified of the results and asked not to donate again. This information is handled with strict confidentiality. Some results are reported to public health departments.

HBV NAT: DNA testing is being considered to reduce window period infections that are currently undetectable by serologic testing for HBs antigen and anti-HBc antibody.

Blood Component Preparation
Most blood is collected as whole blood and then processed into one or more the following components: Red Blood Cells, Plasma and Platelets. Blood is collected into either 450 mL or 500 mL bags containing approximately 63 or 70 mL of anticoagulant-preservative solution, respectively. The anticoagulant is usually either citrate phosphate dextrose (CPD) or citrate phosphate dextrose adenine (CPDA1). CPD is chosen if the Red Blood Cell unit will be enriched with an additive solution. An example of the latter is Adsol (AS-1), which contains saline, adenine, dextrose and mannitol. Additive solutions increase the shelf life of Red Blood Cells from 35 to 42 days.

The most commonly used blood collection bag system is composed of three bags; a primary collection bag containing CPD into which whole blood is drawn and two a satellite bags. Following collection, the triple bag is centrifuged at a slow speed to separate red cells from platelet rich plasma (PRP). The PRP is transferred into the satellite bag. Adsol is added to the RBC bag, which is then clamped, removed sterilely, and stored at 1-6°C for up to 42 days. PRP is then centrifuged a second time at a faster speed to separate platelets and plasma. The supernatant contains platelet poor plasma, which is expressed into the other satellite bag and frozen within either 8 or 24 hours at –18°C. This component is labeled as either Fresh Frozen Plasma (FFP) or 24 hour plasma. The remaining platelet concentrate consists of platelets suspended in approximately 50 mL of plasma. It is allowed to stand at room temperature (20 – 24°C) for one hour and then placed on a platelet rotator for storage up to 5 days at room temperature.

If cryoprecipitate is to be prepared from FFP, the FFP is allowed to freeze for 24 hours and then thawed in a refrigerator. After thawing to a slush stage, FFP is spun in a refrigerated centrifuge to separate the cryoprecipitate from plasma. The supernatant plasma is removed, leaving cryoprecipitate suspended in approximately 15 mL of plasma. The cryoprecipitate is stored frozen at –18°C for up to 12 months. The cryosupernatant or cryo-poor plasma can also be refrozen and stored for up to 12 months.

Blood Component Storage

Blood Component	Shelf Life	Storage Temperature
Red Cells with Adsol	42 days	1-6°C
Platelet Concentrates	5 days	Room temperature
Fresh Frozen Plasma	1 year	-18°C or colder
Cryoprecipitate	1 year	-18°C or colder

Leukocytes can be removed from cellular components by the use of leukocyte reduction filters. Red blood cells can be filtered either immediately after collection, which is called prestorage leukocyte reduction, or at the time of transfusion, which is called bedside filtration. Prestorage leukocyte reduction is preferred because it removes leukocytes before they can release cytokines and ensures better quality control over the filtration process.

AUTOLOGOUS DONATION

Autologous donor programs allow a patient to donate blood for their own use. Autologous transfusion indicates that the blood donor and transfusion recipient are identical. This is the safest possible transfusion a patient can receive and is an excellent option for patients facing elective surgery.

Autologous collections should be used as part of a comprehensive strategy of blood conservation that includes careful attention to the proper indications for transfusion, acceptance of normovolemic anemia and avoidance of excessive blood sampling for diagnostic testing. Autologous donation is a safe procedure, even for very young or elderly patients. Three types of autologous collections are preoperative collection, hemodilution, and intraoperative or postoperative blood salvage

Preoperative Collection
Collection of autologous blood prior to surgery peaked in 1992 at 8% of the United States blood supply and has declined significantly thereafter. The decline has been largely attributed to the increasing safety of the volunteer allogeneic blood supply. Autologous collections have been used most successfully for orthopedic and urologic (radical prostatectomy) surgery. Autologous blood is also beneficial for the patient with alloantibodies to multiple high incidence antigens. Autologous blood should not be collected for surgical or obstetrical procedures, which seldom require transfusion. The ideal patient for autologous donation is one who:

- Has 2 or more weeks before surgery
- Is likely to require blood transfusion during or after surgery
- Has a hemoglobin level greater than 11 g/dL (hematocrit 33%).

Because of the special medical value of autologous collection, blood donor criteria have been relaxed compared to allogeneic donation. The medical director may adjust the hemoglobin criterion higher or lower depending on the clinical circumstances of the donor. There are no age or weight limits. Pediatric donors require more preparation, attention and parental participation.

Some individuals may not be good candidates for autologous donation. Patients taking antihypertensive medications such as beta-blockers may not be able to maintain blood pressure following multiple donations. Autologous blood donation by pregnant women is beneficial only in selected cases such as alloantibodies to multiple or high-incidence antigens, placenta previa, high-risk pregnancy, and bleeding disorders. Patients with severe aortic stenosis, unstable angina, recent myocardial infarction, cyanotic heart disease, cerebrovascular accident, uncontrolled hypertension, active seizure disorder, and bacteremia are usually considered at too high a risk for autologous donation.

In addition to general information about blood donation, autologous donors need information about additional fees charged for autologous services. Because preoperative autologous units require special handling and tracking, most facilities charge an additional autologous fee. Many of these additional charges are not covered by health insurance and are billed to the patient. Medicare covers autologous donation, but some major health insurers do not. Patients also need to be informed that they are responsible for charges even if the unit is not used.

As soon as the surgery date has been scheduled, the attending physician prescribes the number of units to be donated. The patient's physician should request autologous blood collection in writing and the collection site should retain the written order. Requests should include patient's name, the number of units, component, anticipated surgical date, surgical procedure, and the physician's signature.

In order for an autologous program to be effective, a sufficient number of units should be drawn from these patients to minimize the possibility of exposure to allogeneic blood. The underlying principles of autologous blood donation are that red blood cells are donated before elective surgery and sufficient time is allowed for the bone marrow to regenerate all of the donated red cell mass, thereby providing additional red cell volume at the time of surgery. In order to insure that autologous donation is beneficial the following recommendations should be considered:

- Autologous donation should not be ordered unless transfusion is likely.
- Single unit autologous donations should be avoided
- More than 2 weeks should be allowed between the last donation and surgery.

A schedule for donations should be established with the donor. Donations can be made at 72-hour intervals, but one week is preferred. The last donation needs to occur at least one week before the scheduled surgery to allow time for adequate volume repletion prior to the general anesthesia and for all testing of the donated units to be completed.

Each unit of blood donated decreases a patient's hemoglobin by 1g/dL. When a donation is made 2 to 3 weeks before surgery, less than one fourth of the blood loss is regenerated. In order to maximize the benefit of autologous transfusions, sufficient time must be allowed for regenerative erythropoiesis to occur. If not, autologous donation may decrease the patient's preoperative hemoglobin level and place them at higher risk of leaving the hospital more anemic than if they had not donated. Alternatively, the patient may require an allogeneic transfusion.

Iron therapy should be started immediately. Ideally, the requesting physician prescribes supplemental iron even before the first donation to allow maximum time for iron intake. Iron deficiency is frequently the limiting factor for individuals seeking to donate multiple units of blood.

All autologous units must be tested for ABO and Rh. If a unit is to be transfused at a facility other than the collecting facility, it must be tested for all disease markers required by FDA. If a donor tests repeatedly reactive for any marker, then a biohazard label is placed on all of their autologous units. Some blood centers leukocyte reduce all autologous and directed donor RBC units.

Indications for transfusion of autologous units are similar to allogeneic transfusions, and autologous units should not be transfused indiscriminately to an asymptomatic patient merely because it is available. Although autologous blood is the safest form of blood transfusion, adverse reactions can occur. Any transfusion may result in fluid overload. Clerical identification errors can occur, leading to the transfusion of incompatible blood to one and maybe two patients. Bacterial contamination can lead to septic shock.

Hemodilution
Some anesthesiologists hemodilute their patients immediately before surgery. While preparing a patient for surgery, they may withdraw 1 to 2 units of fresh whole blood and replace this volume with IV fluids. The units of blood must be labeled properly and stored at room temperature. They must be reinfused to the patient within 8 hours after collection to prevent deterioration of platelets and coagulation factors. No additional testing is necessary.

This protocol reduces the need to use someone else's blood for transfusion. It also reduces the total red cell mass lost during surgery since the blood is diluted with IV fluids. However, only a limited number of units can be collected this way and not all patients can tolerate such changes in blood volume.

Intra-operative Autologous Blood Collection

Intra-operative collection involves the aspiration, filtration, and reinfusion of shed blood from a clean surgical site or from an extracorporeal circuit. The equipment used for this type of blood salvage varies and may include a wash cycle to remove plasma, activated coagulation factors, and hemolyzed red cells.

Any of the following may be an indication for intraoperative collection:

- Anticipated blood loss is >20% of the patient's estimated blood volume
- More than 10% of patients undergoing the procedure require transfusion
- Average transfusion requirements exceed I unit.

The procedure is most commonly used in cardiac or vascular surgery, orthopedic surgery, selected neurosurgeries, and for trauma patients with penetrating chest wounds.

Certain criteria must be met including:

- Hemoglobin of 12 g/dL or greater
- Absence of clinically significant coronary, pulmonary, renal or liver disease
- Absence of severe hypertension
- Absence of infection or risk of bacteremia

Contraindications are relative and a risk to benefit ratio should be determined for each use. Traditionally, blood is not collected from wounds or sites contaminated with infection, bowel contents, malignant tumor cells, or amniotic fluid. Aspiration of topical hemostatic agents, wound irrigants, and antibiotics not licensed for parenteral use should also be avoided.

Post-operative Autologous Blood Collection

Shed blood can only be transfused to the patient from which it was collected and procedures must ensure proper identification of the unit to the patient. The unit must be labeled with the patient's name, identification number, date and time of collection, expiration date and the statement "For Autologous Use Only". If it is stored in the Blood Bank, it must be handled like any other autologous unit except that disease testing may be waived. The unit should be stored at room temperature for up to 6 hours or at 1 to 6°C for up to 24 hours if storage begins within 4 hours of collection.

DIRECTED BLOOD DONATIONS

Directed donations are units of blood directly solicited from family or friends by the intended recipient. Some patients anticipating elective surgery prefer to receive blood donated by relatives or friends, even though directed donations have not been proven to be safer than those from the community blood supply. Laws in many states have been established which protect the patient's right to request directed donation.

Physicians initiate the order for directed donation of blood at a patient's request. The order must specify the number of units needed, transfusion date(s), and patient's ABO and Rh type. The patient should instruct his/her directed donors to donate a few days to a few weeks before the anticipated transfusion to allow adequate time for donor scheduling, blood collection, test completion, and shipping.

Directed donors must have a blood type that is compatible with the recipient and meet the same donor requirements as volunteer donors. The same tests are performed on directed units as volunteer units. Generally, donors give blood only once every 8 weeks. To reduce the number of donors a patient is exposed to, special arrangements can be made to have some designated donors give more frequently. These frequent donors must continue to meet all other donor requirements each time they donate.

Specific directed donor policies vary with institution. Only acceptable, ABO and Rh compatible directed donor units are reserved for a patient. Units that are ABO and Rh incompatible are either not drawn or released to general inventory. Most facilities reserve directed donor units only for a specified time, such as 5 days after the scheduled transfusion date or 1 week before the unit expires. After this time, they may be released to general stock and used on someone else to prevent unnecessary waste, although some institutions will not use them for other patients because of concerns that a directed donation may not be as safe as a volunteer non-directed donation. If the anticipated date of transfusion changes, the physician should notify the Blood Bank immediately so that the reservation time is extended. Directed donor units are not routinely frozen to extend storage. Instead, additional donors are recruited.

Because directed donor units require extra handling and tracking, they usually cost more than regular volunteer units. These charges are billed whether or not the unit is transfused. Directed donations, like autologous units, may not be covered by health insurance reimbursement. Patients seeking directed donation should be informed of this possibility.

Indications for Directed Donation include:
1. Indications for autologous blood cited above.
2. Bone marrow donor components after transplant.
3. Family red blood cells for rare blood groups.

Directed donations may cause complications such as: maternal sensitization to paternal antigens, sensitization to HLA antigens, and the development of graft versus host disease. Men are advised against donating for their female sexual partners of child bearing age since this could increase the risk of hemolytic disease of the newborn in future pregnancies. Potential bone marrow donors should not donate blood pre-transplantation for the recipient because transfusion may lead to HLA sensitization and subsequent bone marrow graft rejection. Relatives should not donate plasma for a coagulation factor deficient patient if they have the same coagulation factor deficiency. Recipients receiving cellular blood components from first-degree relatives are at increased risk of developing graft versus host disease. Thus, all directed donor units of whole blood, red blood cells, platelets, and granulocytes must be irradiated.

APHERESIS

Apheresis employs an automated cell separator that harvests a specific blood component by centrifugal force. It involves a multi-step process that includes:
- Removal of whole blood from a donor or patient
- Separation of whole blood into components such as red cells, plasma, platelets or white cells
- Retention of the specific component needed
- Return of the unneeded recombined components to the donor.

Apheresis takes 1 to 2 hours to complete. During this time the donor or patient is connected by 1 or 2 IV lines to a sterile set of collecting and infusion bags. This closed system eliminates the risks of bacterial contamination and of returning the wrong blood to the donor.

Red cells may be collected by apheresis. Two allogeneic or autologous red cell units may be removed every 16 weeks. Volume depletion is minimized with saline infusion and the procedure is limited to individuals who are larger and have higher hematocrits (>40%) than current minimum standards for whole blood donors.

Plasmapheresis involves the separation of fresh plasma from 1 to 1.2 L of whole blood from a single donor, depending on the donor's weight. This component is usually processed into Fresh Frozen Plasma or Cryoprecipitate. Its larger volume (usually equivalent to 2 units FFP) can be used by one patient to reduce donor exposures or can be aliquoted to benefit several patients.

Plateletpheresis is the collection of platelets from a single donor and is often called single donor platelets. Donors should not take aspirin within 36 hours of donation. Blood pumped from one arm passes through a blood cell separator centrifugation system that collects platelets and returns plasma and red cells to the donor's other arm. Between 4000 and 5000 mL of blood are processed over 1.5 to 2 hours. A single donor platelet concentrate contains >3.0 X 10^{11} platelets suspended in approximately 200 mL of plasma, which is the equivalent of 6 to 8 random donor platelet concentrates. They can be stored up to 5 days at room temperature.

Because red cells and plasma are returned, a plateletpheresis donor can give more frequently than a whole blood donor; once or twice a week. This procedure is ideal for collecting platelets from special donors such as directed donor, platelet crossmatch compatible or HLA-matched.

Single donor apheresis platelets contain fewer than 5 x 106 white blood cells and are considered to be leukocyte reduced. Additional leukocyte reduction filtration is not necessary. Rh negative patients do not need Rh immune globulin after transfusion of Rh positive apheresis platelets because they contain so few red blood cells.

CHAPTER 5:
Informed Consent,
Alternatives and Risks of Transfusion

There are two major legal issues pertaining to the clinical aspects of blood transfusion:

1. Avoidance of transfusions that are not medically indicated
2. Documentation in the medical chart that there is a valid indication for transfusion.

Prior to the mid 1980s, a signed informed consent specific for blood transfusion was rarely obtained. Instead, hospitals took the position that informed consent for blood transfusion was implicitly granted when a patient agreed to undergo a medical or surgical procedure or even to be admitted to the hospital. This interpretation of adequate consent for transfusion began to be questioned in the mid 1980s with the recognition of transfusion associated HIV.

After the advent of HIV, transfusion was perceived as carrying an excessive risk relative to other medical events. In 1986, the American Association of Blood Banks recommended that patients receiving nonemergent transfusions should be informed of the risks and benefits of blood and blood products and consent to their use. Informed consent for transfusion is a standard for accreditation required by the Joint Commission. Such consent can either be documented by a progress note in the medical chart, a signed consent form, or both.

Informed consent should be obtained prior to all blood and blood product transfusions, except in emergency situations. If a patient is incompetent by age or mental status, and if the patient's wishes regarding transfusion are not known, consent should be sought from the parent or legal guardian.

Informed consent should include the following elements:

1. The patient must be competent.
2. The treating physician, or the treating team, who decides that the transfusion is necessary should obtain consent.
3. The procedure must be explained in terms and language that the patient understands.
4. The patient should be informed of the risks, potential benefits, and alternatives to transfusion as well as the possible consequences of declining transfusion.
5. The patient must have the opportunity to ask questions.
6. The patient must have the right to accept or refuse the transfusion.
7. The discussion must be documented.

When applicable, the consent and discussion should occur well in advance of any elective procedure, so that alternatives may be obtained if the patient desires. Alternatives to allogeneic transfusion include:

*   Autologous donation
*   Directed donation
*   Blood conservation techniques
*   Erythropoietin and iron therapy

A discussion of risks should weigh the risks of receiving the transfusion against the risk of withholding transfusion for each individual patient. Today, the blood supply is extremely safe due to extensive donor screening and laboratory testing. However, a small number of trans-fused patients experience adverse transfusion reactions. An adverse reaction is defined as any unfavorable event that occurs during or after a transfusion. The cellular or fluid portions of the blood, anticoagulant-preservative solution, metabolic by-products, and circulating or contami-nant microorganisms may cause adverse reactions. The estimated risks and etiologies of the most common transfusion reactions are listed below. Risk is expressed per unit of transfused blood rather than per patient. In this way, a patient's actual risk can more accurately be esti-mated by multiplying the per unit risk times the number of units transfused.

Immunologic Risks

Reaction	Etiology	# Cases per Unit Transfused
Urticaria	Ab to donor proteins	1:4,000
Anaphylaxis	Ab to donor IgA	1:30,000
Febrile	Ab to donor WBCs	1:1000
TRALI	Ab to recipient WBCs	1:5,000
Wrong patient transfused	Human error	1:38,000
Hemolytic, acute	Ab to donor RBCs	1:100,000
Hemolytic, fatal	ABO incompatibility	1:1,800,000
Alloimmunization	Ab to donor cells	1:200
Graft vs Host Disease	HLA incompatibility	1:1,000,000

Today, TRALI and patient identification errors cause more transfusion related fatalities than HCV or HIV-1. The only way to prevent these errors from happening is meticulous attention to the patient identification protocol and the introduction of technological advances such as bar coded wristbands.

Hepatitis C and HIV-1 viruses have been almost completely eliminated from the blood supply. These improvements have occurred largely through more comprehensive donor history screening, technological advances in infectious disease testing, and development of virus inactivation techniques for coagulation factor concentrates. Since the risks of transfu-sion transmitted infection are currently very low, it is difficult to accurately quantitate them. Consequently, risk estimates have been obtained with mathematical modeling techniques applied to data sets obtained from infectious disease testing of blood donors or follow-up investigations of selected transfusion recipients. The current estimated risks of transfusion transmitted infection, expressed per unit of blood received, are given in the following table.

Estimated Transfusion Risk

Infection	Per Unit Risk Estimate
HIV-1	1 in 2,000,000
HIV-2	None
HTLV-I/II	1 in 2,990,000
HBV	1 in 205,000 - 408,000
HCV	1 in 1,935,000
West Nile Virus	None
Bacterial contamination of apheresis platelets	1 in 75,000

For the most important transfusion transmissible agents, Human Immunodeficiency Virus

(HIV) and Hepatitis C virus (HCV), the per unit risk is the same for each type of blood component transfused (i.e. red cells, platelets, FFP, cryoprecipitate). In contrast, for Human T cell Lymphotropic Virus Types I and II (HTLV-I/II) there is no risk of transmission from non-cellular blood products such as FFP or cryoprecipitate, since HTLV is highly leukocyte-associated.

It is unlikely that transfusion transmitted diseases will ever be completely eliminated for the following reasons:

- Some high risk individuals continue to donate
- Infected donors may be asymptomatic
- Tests are not 100% sensitive
- Human errors cannot be completely eliminated.

A nucleic acid or serological test may not become positive during the early stages of infection, known as the window period. For example, an individual exposed to HIV will not have a detectable viral load for at least 11 days following infection and antibody will not be detectable for 22 days. If an individual were to donate blood during this window period, their transfused blood components would be capable of transmitting HIV infection.

Platelets are stored up to five days at room temperature under aerobic conditions, which are ideal conditions for bacterial growth. Bacterial contamination has become one of the major risk factors to patient safety.

CHAPTER 6:
Blood Administration

To help ensure the benefits and safety of a blood transfusion, the appropriate blood component must be ordered and it must be properly infused.

PREPARATION FOR TRANSFUSION

The physician initiates the request for blood by a written order in the patient's medical record. If informed consent has not already been obtained, the physician should explain the risks and alternatives of transfusion to the recipient or responsible family member and document this discussion in the medical record.

The written order is forwarded to the Transfusion Service. If needed, a blood specimen is drawn for compatibility testing. It is important to specify the time of transfusion and any special instructions such as the need for CMV negative or irradiated products. Routine testing takes about 1 hour to complete and some products require extra preparation time.

Because blood contains living cells and has special storage requirements, nurses should not send for the product until an IV has been started, necessary equipment is gathered, and both patient and staff are ready to begin the transfusion. If the recipient requires medication to prevent an allergic or febrile reaction, it should be given immediately prior to transfusion.

The transfusion should be started as soon as the blood arrives on the floor. If it will be delayed the product should be returned to the Blood Bank for proper storage and later reissue.

TRANSFUSION EQUIPMENT

Blood Infusion Sets
Blood components must be filtered during transfusion to remove clots and small clumps of platelets and white blood cells that form during collection and storage. Standard blood infusion sets contain 170 - 260 micron filters. Smaller component sets with in-line filters for plasma, platelets, and red cell aliquots are also available.

The manufacturer provides instructions for priming and use on the infusion set package. Blood sets should not be piggy-backed into other lines if this can be avoided. If they must be piggy-backed, the Injection port closest to the IV line should be used and the primary IV line shut off. Straight-type sets are primed directly with the blood component. Y-type sets can be primed with blood or Normal Saline. Usually, a new set is used for each component transfused. If 2 units are to be given consecutively and they are ABO compatible with one another, one set may be used for both as long as they are infused within 4 hours.

Needles and Catheters
Needle size depends on the size and integrity of a patient's vein. An 18-gauge needle is standard, but a needle or catheter as small as 23-gauge can be used for transfusion if necessary. The smaller the gauge, the slower is the flow rate and the higher is the risk of clotting. Care must be taken to avoid excessive pressure and resulting hemolysis when very narrow devices are used. Diluting red cells with saline or asking the Transfusion Service to split a unit and giving only half at a time may help if the flow rate is too slow.

Leukocyte Removal Filters
Special bedside filters may be provided by the Transfusion Service when pre-storage leukocyte-reduced red cells or platelets are not available. Red cell and platelet filters do not use

the same technology for leukocyte removal and are not interchangeable. Some are designed to attach to standard infusion sets; others come with a set already attached. Most leukocyte-removing filters are designed for gravity drip use and have special priming requirements, so it is essential to check the manufacturer's directions before use.

IV Pumps
Mechanical pumps may be useful for controlling the very slow infusion rates required by neonatal and pediatric patients, but care is needed to avoid hemolysis. Only pumps specifically approved for blood transfusion should be used. Some pumps can be used with standard infusion sets; others require special software.

Pressure Bags
Pressure bags are needed only in emergency situations when blood must be transfused rapidly, such as 5 minutes per unit. The bag should be inflated only until blood flow through the drip chamber is continuous, about 200 mm Hg. Pressure approaching 300 mm Hg may cause the red cells to Iyse and the blood bag seams to split.

Blood Warmers
Blood warmers are used to prevent cardiac arrhythmia associated with the rapid infusion of large volumes of cold blood. Specific indications include:

- Adults receiving blood at a rate in excess of 100 mL per minute
- Children receiving blood over 15 mL/kg/hour
- Patients with clinically significant cold agglutinins
- Rapid infusion of blood through central lines.

Blood should not be warmed to a temperature that causes hemolysis. Only temperature-controlled and monitored in-line devices are acceptable for use, and some require special software. The blood warmer must have a visible thermometer and, ideally, an audible alarm. The warmer should be set up according to the manufacturers' directions and its temperature checked periodically during use.

IV Solutions and Medications
Normal Saline (0.9% sodium chloride) can be added to blood, but drugs and medications must never be added. Compatible plasma or 5% Albumin, and Plasma Protein Fraction can be added to blood following approval by the patient's physician. Isotonic electrolyte solutions that do not contain calcium may mix with blood if the FDA approves the solution for such use or if there is adequate documentation of safety. Some solutions should not contact blood in the bag or tubing. Solutions containing glucose (e.g. 5% dextrose) may cause red cells to aggregate and Iyse and those containing calcium (e.g. Ringer's Lactate) may cause blood to clot.

CONFIRMING PATIENT AND DONOR IDENTITY

When blood arrives on the nursing unit, the patient's medical record should be checked to verify the physician's request and to assess special transfusion instructions that may impact patient care. Then 2 responsible individuals must confirm the identity and compatibility of the donor and recipient. This is a 3-step process:

1. By reading aloud to one another from the blood bag label and the attached transfusion form, two nurses or physicians verify that:
   a) Patient name and ID number is identical on all paperwork.
   b) Donor number is identical on all paperwork.
   c) The correct blood component product was received.

        d)   ABO & Rh type of the patient and donor are compatible.

        e)   Expiration date & time has not passed.

        f)   Color or appearance of blood is normal.

        g)   Special instructions, if noted, are carried out.

2. At the patient's bedside, these same 2 individuals verify that the patient's name and ID number are identical on the patient's hospital ID band and the blood bank transfusion Form

3. These same 2 individuals then sign the transfusion form and immediately start the transfusion.

Transfusion should not begin unless this identity check is accurate and complete. Discrepant information must be resolved with the Transfusion Service beforehand. If the unit cannot be started immediately after the identity check, all 3 steps should be repeated. The compatibility tag should remain attached to the bag during transfusion; the transfusion form may be placed in the chart or on a clipboard in the patient's room until the transfusion is complete.

MONITORING THE PATIENT DURING TRANSFUSION

Patients must be observed during transfusion for signs and symptoms of an adverse transfusion reaction. This includes monitoring vital signs and general well being and documenting the results in the medical record. Because life-threatening reactions can occur within minutes, a physician or nurse should remain at the bedside for 5 to 15 minutes after the transfusion is started.

Baseline vital signs such as temperature, pulse, blood pressure and respiration rate should be documented immediately prior to spiking the bag and starting the transfusion. Comparison values are recorded again approximately 15 minutes after starting the transfusion and then periodically during the transfusion.

Any change in the patient's clinical status during or following a transfusion or an inadequate response to transfusion should be carefully evaluated. Because some reactions are delayed, patients should be monitored up to 1 hour post transfusion.

INFUSION RATES

Packed red blood cells can be diluted with 0.9% NaCl to decrease viscosity and improve flow rate. Adsol units usually do not require further dilution, because they have already been diluted by the addition of preservative. Red cells should be infused through an IV catheter and a standard 170 micron filter at a rate of 2 mL/minute for the first 15 minutes. The recipient should be observed for evidence of a transfusion reaction during this time period. If no adverse effects occur, the rate can be increased to 4 mL/minute for nonemergent transfusions. An infusion rate of 17mL/min allows an entire unit of blood to be transfused in 30 minutes. The usual recommended time period ranges between 1.5 and 2 hours per unit. The maximum time period allowed for infusion of a single unit of blood is 4 hours. In emergency situations, the infusion rate is not as well established. Infusion rates greater than 60mL/min are dangerous, and infusion rates greater than 100mL/min are associated with cardiac arrest. External pressure devices can be used to increase the rate of infusion. The pressure exerted should not exceed 300 mm Hg. Blood pressure cuffs should not be used because they apply pressure non-uniformly and can cause leakage.

Platelets are transfused through platelet filters at a rate which allows a pool of random donor platelets or a single donor platelet to be transfused within 30 to 60 minutes. FFP is usually transfused through a standard blood filter at a rate of 30 to 60 minutes per bag. Cryoprecipitate is infused through a standard blood filter at a rate of 4 to 10 mL/minute. At this rate, a pool of 10 bags can be infused in approximately 30 minutes.

TRANSFUSION FOLLOW-UP

After the blood component is transfused, the transfusion form must be completed and placed in the patient's medical record. The blood component (e.g. red cells, platelets, etc), donor number, and transfusion time are recorded on the hospital transfusion record. Observations and/or patient responses during transfusion are charted in the nursing notes. There must be enough information documented in the medical record to show that protocols were followed in the event there is a reaction or complication.

The empty blood bag and its attached administration set are considered to be biologically contaminated waste and should be disposed of according to hospital policy. If a transfusion reaction occurs, the bag and set should be sealed in a plastic bag and returned to the Transfusion Service for the reaction investigation.

Transfusion Delays
If the start of a transfusion is delayed after a unit of Red Blood Cells has been issued, the unit can be returned to inventory if it has not remained at room temperature for more than 30 minutes. The Red Blood Cell unit's temperature will usually not exceed 10°C for at least the first 30 minutes at room temperature. If a unit remains at room temperature for longer periods of time, glucose and ATP might become depleted and any contaminating bacteria might begin to proliferate.

CHAPTER 7:
Transfusion Reactions

Every year more than 5 million individuals in the United States are transfused with allogeneic and autologous blood components. In spite of extensive donor screening and laboratory testing, a small number of transfused patients experience adverse transfusion reactions. An adverse reaction is defined as any unfavorable event that occurs during or after a transfusion. The cellular or fluid portions of the blood, anticoagulant-preservative solution, metabolic by-products, and circulating or contaminant microorganisms may cause adverse reactions. The estimated risks and etiologies of the most common transfusion reactions were summarized in Chapter 5.

When an adverse transfusion reaction occurs, medical, nursing and laboratory personnel must be prepared to recognize and treat them. Because the signs and symptoms of different types of adverse reactions overlap and their severity can vary considerably, all transfusions must be carefully monitored and stopped as soon as symptoms of a reaction appear. Early recognition is the key to minimizing serious complications. Signs and symptoms of a transfusion reaction include:

Fever (>1°C, 2°F)	Warmth at infusion site	Wheezing or rales
Rigors	Myalgia	Coughing
Hives, rash or itching	Chest or back pain	Dyspnea
Facial flushing	Hypotension	Cyanosis
Headache	Oliguria or anuria	Pulmonary edema
Nausea	Abnormal bleeding or DIC	Hemoglobinuria
Uneasy feeling	Jaundice	Shock

NURSING ACTION

For any acute reaction other than hives, the nursing or medical staff should take the following action:

1. Stop the transfusion immediately and disconnect the entire infusion set from the needle or catheter

2. Keep the IV line open with a slow drip of Normal Saline, using a new infusion set.

3. Check the blood bag label and paperwork against the patient's ID band to confirm that the patient received the correct unit.

4. Notify the attending physician so that treatment, if necessary, can begin immediately.

5. Take vital signs every 15 minutes until the patient is stable.

6. Notify the Transfusion Service & describe the signs and symptoms of the reaction.

7. Send the following items on a STAT basis:

    • Completed transfusion reaction form

    • Blood component bag with attached infusion set & IV fluids.

    • Post transfusion blood sample

    • Post-transfusion urine specimen

LABORATORY RESPONSE

The Transfusion Service staff will immediately determine whether hemolysis has occurred. If possible, testing should be performed by someone other than the person who completed the original testing. Laboratory evaluation of a suspected hemolytic reaction can follow a hierarchic approach. For example, testing may be divided into Tier One and Tier Two. First Tier testing is designed to detect hemolysis, but cannot differentiate immune from other causes of hemolysis. Negative first tier testing rules out hemolysis. Second tier testing is performed if first tier testing indicates that hemolysis occurred. It is intended to establish the diagnosis of immune hemolysis.

Tier One Testing

Tier one testing encompasses :

- Clerical check for procedural or identification errors
- Visual check of post-transfusion plasma for hemolysis
- Comparison of blood types on pre and post-transfusion specimens
- Direct antiglobulin test on post-reaction sample

The detailed steps include:

1) Inspecting the label on the transfusion tag and blood bag and all other records to detect an error in identifying the patient or the unit of blood.

2) Checking the appearance of the blood bag, administration set and saline for discoloration or hemolysis.

3) Comparing patient's pre and post transfusion specimens for proper identification.

4) Visually inspecting pre and post transfusion plasma for hemoglobin or bilirubin.

5) If hemolysis is observed in the post transfusion specimen, requesting another specimen to rule out mechanical hemolysis.

6) Performing an ABO & Rh type on the post transfusion specimen and comparing the results to the pre transfusion specimen results.

7) Performing a DAT on the post transfusion specimen. If the post DAT is positive, performing a DAT on the pre transfusion specimen.

Hemolysis in the post-transfusion sample, but not the pre-transfusion sample is suspicious of a hemolytic transfusion reaction. As little as 20 mg/dL of hemoglobin will make the plasma appear pink, while 50 mg/dL or more will make it appear red. This degree of hemoglobinemia corresponds to the hemolysis of 4 to 10 mL of RBCs. Hemolysis in both samples suggests that some other explanation must be sought (see nonimmune hemolysis section below).

If the DAT is positive on the post-reaction specimen, a pre-transfusion reaction sample should be tested for comparison. If the post transfusion DAT is positive, but the pre-transfusion DAT is negative a hemolytic transfusion reaction is possible. Since circulating antibody or complement coated red cells may be rapidly cleared, the DAT may be negative especially if the specimen was drawn several hours after the suspected reaction. If incompatible transfused cells have been partially destroyed, the DAT may have a mixed field appearance. The DAT will be positive if at least 10% of a patient's red cells are coated with IgG.

If both the pre and post-transfusion DAT are positive, the test is not helpful in diagnosis of a hemolytic transfusion reaction, because the DAT may be the result of:

- Autoimmune hemolytic anemia
- Benign red cell autoantibody
- Drug sensitization
- Intravenous immune globulin (IVIg) infusion
- RhIg administration
- Transfusion of a DAT positive donor red cell unit.

No further investigation is necessary if:

1) The clerical checks match each other.
2) No hemolysis is observed.
3) Pre and post transfusion blood types are the same.
4) DAT is negative.

In this case, the Transfusion Reaction form is signed by the Clinical Laboratory Scientist and left for Pathologist review & interpretation. After the form has been signed, one copy is placed in the medical record and a second copy is kept in the Transfusion Service.

Tier Two Testing
If any part of Tier One testing is positive or the patient's medical condition strongly suggests a hemolytic reaction, then Tier Two testing is undertaken.

1) Repeat ABO & Rh type, antibody screen and DAT on the pre and post transfusion specimens and blood from the unit in question.
2) Perform major and minor antiglobulin crossmatches on the pre and post blood specimens.
3) If results indicate a hemolytic reaction, immediately notify the patient's physician and a pathologist.
4) Test the patient's first post transfusion urine sample with a dipstick for hemoglobin. If positive, perform a microscopic urinalysis to rule out the presence of intact RBCs.
5) Measure patient's post transfusion hemoglobin and compare it to the pre transfusion value.
6) Order a pre and post transfusion haptoglobin level.
7) Order a pre and post transfusion total and direct bilirubin and repeat in 4 to 6 hours.
8) Consult the pathologist to determine if additional tests are warranted.
9) If bacterial contamination is suspected, the following should be done:
   a) Notify the patient's physician and the pathologist immediately.
   b) Perform a gram stain on blood from the blood bag in question.
   c) Ask Microbiology to set up aerobic and anaerobic blood cultures on blood from the bag (not from a segment) and any IV solution hanging with the unit.
   d Ask the physician to order 2 sets of blood cultures on the patient.
10) If Transfusion Related Acute Lung Injury (TRALI) is suspected
   a) Complete Tier One testing
   b) Consult the pathologist to determine if a granulocyte antibody should be ordered on the patient.
   c) Notify the Blood Center that supplied the unit so that they can:

   i)   Review donor history.
   ii) Perform a granulocyte antibody on the donor's plasma.
   iii) Defer the donor from future donations if TRALI is confirmed.
   d)   Notify the FDA through MedWatch.

If ABO and Rh typing on the pre and post-reaction samples do not agree, there has been an error in patient or sample identification or testing. If so, another patient's blood sample may have been drawn and incorrectly labeled, making it imperative to check the records of all specimens received at approximately the same time. If the donor blood type is not the same ABO type as the bag label, then an error has occurred in either labeling or processing of the unit.

If hemolysis is observed in the blood bag, red blood cells may have been hemolyzed because the unit was improperly transported, stored, warmed or mixed with a hypotonic IV solution.

In a hemolytic reaction, DAT may be positive and antibody screen negative. In this situation, a red cell eluate can be used for antibody identification.

Pre and post crossmatches should be performed, including the antiglobulin phase, to detect an antibody to a low frequency antigen or an error in pretransfusion testing. Whenever possible, the pre-transfusion crossmatch should be repeated with cells from a retained segment. If an incompatibility is found, a second crossmatch should be performed with the pre-transfusion serum and donor unit red cells to see if incompatibility was present prior to transfusion.

- If both pre and post-reaction crossmatches are incompatible, an error was almost certainly made during pre-transfusion testing. The donor specimen used for the original crossmatch may have been taken from a different unit or the patient's antibody screen was incorrectly read as negative.

- If the crossmatch is incompatible with the post-reaction specimen but compatible with the pre-reaction specimen, anamnestic recall of antibody may have occurred. Antibody may have developed to red cells transfused in the preceding few days. Less likely, antibody may have been present in the transfused blood component and passively transfused.

Once an antibody has been identified, it is helpful to antigen type red cells from the transfused units to determine how many units were incompatible. The potential severity of hemolysis can be estimated from the number of antigen positive units transfused.

Acute Hemolytic Reactions without Detectable Antibody
Occasionally, a severe hemolytic reaction occurs, but the serological workup does not detect a red cell antibody. Sometimes the use of antibody enhancement techniques such as Polybrene, polyethylene glycol (PEG) or enzyme treated red cells reveals the causative antibody, which usually has specificity for C, E, e, S, Jk^a, or Jk^b. However, in many cases these techniques are not helpful. HLA antibodies may be responsible for some of these hemolytic reactions. HLA A28, B7 and B17 are present on red cells and are termed Bg^c, Bg^b and Bg^a, respectively. Bg antigens are excluded from antibody screening cells. If one of these patients requires additional urgent transfusion, the best option is to provide phenotypically matched red cell units.

Reporting of Adverse Reactions
- A Sentinel Event must be reported to the hospital's Risk Management department.
- If a transfusion related fatality occurs, the Transfusion Service must notify the FDA's Center for Biologics Evaluation and Research (CBER) within 24 hours and file a written report within 7 days.

- The blood collection facility should be notified if any adverse reaction is suspected to be due an attribute of the donor or a problem with the collection, processing, or shipment of the blood component.

TYPES OF TRANSFUSION REACTIONS

Clinical and laboratory personnel must be familiar with the different types of transfusion reactions so that the most appropriate testing and treatment are instituted. For this discussion, reactions have been classified as early or late onset. Early onset reactions occur during or within a few hours of transfusion, while late onset reactions occur days to months following transfusion.

EARLY ONSET REACTIONS

Allergic Reactions

Simple allergic reactions are the second most common type of transfusion complication. Allergic reactions occur most commonly after the transfusion of components containing large volumes of plasma such as fresh frozen plasma, plasma frozen within 24 hours, single donor platelets or pooled random donor platelet concentrates. Transfusion of red blood cells is less commonly associated with allergic reactions because they contain so little plasma.

Etiology: Allergic reactions are attributed to soluble substances in donor plasma (e.g. food allergens, drugs or ethylene oxide) which react with IgE antibody bound to basophils or mast cells in the recipient's blood. This interaction results in the release of C3a, C5a, histamine, prostaglandin D2, leukotrienes C and D4 and a variety of other cytokines. These substances produce an immediate type hypersensitivity reaction by increasing vascular permeability, promoting bronchial smooth muscle contractions, and stimulating mucus secretion by nasal and bronchial glands. Histamine release causes hives, itching, and rarely, laryngeal edema.

Symptoms: Hives (urticaria) or other rash (erythema), itching (pruritis), and wheezing are most common. Allergic reactions can occur during or up to 3 hours post-transfusion. The shorter the time interval between the start of the transfusion and the onset of the allergic reaction, the more severe the reaction. In more severe reactions, anxiety, dyspnea, palpitations, fever and chills may accompany urticaria.

Consequences: Allergic reactions are not usually dangerous, but they do cause discomfort and anxiety. Urticaria is not a manifestation of a hemolytic reaction, so it is not usually necessary to discontinue the transfusion.

Lab Data: No laboratory testing is necessary.

Treatment:
1. Slow the rate of transfusion for 15 to 30 minutes.
2. Give an antihistamine to ease discomfort.
3. Monitor carefully because urticaria could be the first sign of a more serious allergic reaction.
4. If the only symptom is skin rash or hives and the symptoms resolve within 30 minutes of treatment, the transfusion can be resumed.

Prevention: Patients who have had 2 or more allergic reactions benefit from oral or parenteral prophylactic treatment with diphenhydramine one hour prior to transfusion and at the start of transfusion. If reactions continue, cellular products can be washed to remove residual plasma containing the soluble allergens. Corticosteroids may be necessary in severe, repetitive cases.

Anaphylactic Reactions
Anaphylactic reactions can be associated with almost any type of blood component and are life-threatening.

Etiology: Absolute IgA deficiency (<0.05 mg/dL) or an IgA subclass deficiency puts a patient at higher risk of having an anaphylactic reaction. Approximately 1 in 1200 people are IgA deficient. Such persons may form IgE antibodies against IgA. When anti-IgA antibody binds to IgA in transfused plasma, complement is activated and severe anaphylaxis can occur.

Although IgA deficiency is the most well known cause of anaphylactic reactions, other causes have also been reported.
- The recipient may have preformed antibodies to transfused allergens, drugs or chemicals.
- Bedside leukoreduction of components for patients receiving ACE inhibitors
- Transfusion of plasma or platelets to patients with Chido or Rogers antibodies
- Accumulation of bioactive lipids, CD40 ligand and cytokines in stored products
- Passive transfer of IgE antibodies or high concentrations of histamine.
- Haptoglobin deficiency

In many cases the cause of the anaphylactic reaction is not identified.

Symptoms: Sudden onset of flushing and hypertension followed by hypotension, tachycardia, widespread edema, laryngeal edema, bronchospasm, shock, and sometimes GI symptoms such as abdominal cramping, nausea, vomiting, and diarrhea can occur within minutes of starting the transfusion.

Consequences: Potentially fatal due to shock or respiratory failure. Early recognition and treatment are critical

Lab Data: TierOne testing should be performed to rule out a hemolytic reaction. No evidence of RBC serological incompatibility will be found in an anaphylactic reaction. IgA deficiency is diagnosed by measuring quantitative immunoglobulin levels on a pretransfusion specimen. Unfortunately, most nephelometric methods for measuring IgA have a lower limit of detection of 5 mg/dL, which is not sensitive enough to diagnose absolute IgA deficiency. A measureable amount of IgA, rules out an absolute deficiency, which practically excludes the likelihood of an anti-IgA mediated anaphylactic reaction. If IgA is deficient, serum can be sent to a reference laboratory for anti-IgA antibody determination.

Treatment:
1. When an anaphylactic reaction is recognized, the transfusion must be stopped immediately and not restarted.
2. The patient should receive airway management and supportive care. Blood pressure and volume should be maintained with crystalloid infusions.
3. The attending physician may need to prescribe medications to treat hypotension and bronchospasm.

Prevention: Patients with a history of anaphylactic reactions or IgA deficiency with documented anti-IgA antibody should receive only washed red blood cells and platelets. If plasma is needed, it must be obtained from a known IgA deficient donor.

Febrile Nonhemolytic Reactions
Febrile reactions are the most common type of transfusion reaction reported to the Blood Bank. Because their symptoms of fever and chills also occur with acute hemolytic reactions, it is essential to evaluate all such reactions immediately.

Etiology: Most febrile reactions that occur during transfusion of red blood cells are caused by the interaction of leukocyte antibodies in the recipient's plasma with donor leukocytes, stimulating the release of pro-inflammatory cytokines such as interleukin-1 (IL-1), interleukin-6 (IL-6) and tumor necrosis factor alpha (TNF). Patients who have had multiple prior transfusions or pregnancies are more likely to have these antibodies. Two thirds of these antibodies have HLA specificity, while one third are specific for platelet or granulocyte antigens. Antibodies usually reach detectable levels within 1 to 2 weeks after transfusion and are often transient. The transient nature of these antibodies may explain why only 1 in 7 patients experience repeat febrile reactions.

At least 2 mechanisms are responsible for febrile reactions to platelet transfusions. Approximately 95% of reactions are caused by cytokines that accumulate in the platelet concentrate during storage. Most of these cytokines do not reach detectable levels until day 3 of storage and may reach high levels by day 5. Transfusion of high levels of these cytokines produces fever. The second mechanism that is responsible for 5% of platelet associated febrile reaction is the interaction of donor leukocytes with anti-leukocyte antibodies in recipient plasma, similar to febrile reactions induced by red cells.

Symptoms: A febrile reaction is defined as an increase in temperature >1°C above the pre-transfusion temperature either during or up to several hours after the transfusion. Fever may persist for 8 to 12 hours. Chills may precede the fever or occur up to 30 minutes after the onset of fever. In some patients, headache, flushing, or tachycardia may accompany fever and chills. Patients who are febrile at the onset of transfusion or have been febrile in the preceding 24 hours, are more prone to febrile reactions.

Consequences: It is important to recognize and report febrile reactions because they may be the first indication of a septic or hemolytic transfusion reaction. A febrile reaction, by itself, is not usually serious, although the patient will have discomfort.

Lab Data:

1. A transfusion reaction work-up should be initiated to rule out a hemolytic or septic reaction.
2. A clerical check should be performed to determine whether the patient received the correct unit. A lavender top tube of blood should be sent to the laboratory.
3. The Transfusion Service should perform Tier One testing.
5. If no clerical error has occurred, the plasma is not red or pink, and the DAT is negative, an acute hemolytic reaction is unlikely and it can be assumed that a febrile reaction occurred.

Treatment:

The transfusion should be discontinued, but the IV line kept open. Medication is usually not required for mild febrile reactions. Antipyretics can be given to relieve moderate to severe symptoms. Acetaminophen is preferred over aspirin. Diphenhydramine is not effective in reducing temperature, but can be given to alleviate chills. Meperidine (Demerol) may be helpful in treating rigors.

Prevention: Only 1 in 7 patients experiencing a febrile nonhemolytic reaction will have another reaction at their next transfusion. If a 2nd reaction does occur, leukocyte-reduced RBCs and platelets should be requested.

The best way to prevent severe febrile reactions is to use prestorage leukocyte reduced single donor platelets. Bedside leukocyte reduction of platelets does not reduce the incidence of febrile reactions. If a patient continues to have febrile reactions to leukocyte reduced single donor platelets, it may be helpful to remove plasma from the platelet unit immediately prior to transfusion. Alternatively, platelets can be washed. Both plasma reduction and washing may activate platelets and decrease their hemostatic effectiveness.

If a patient continues to experience febrile reactions even after receiving leukocyte reduced blood components, it may be necessary to pre-medicate them with 650 mg acetaminophen and 25 mg of diphenhydramine. Pre-medication should be used judiciously since it may mask the early signs and symptoms of a hemolytic reaction.

Acute Hemolytic Transfusion Reaction (AHTR)
Today, it is estimated that 1 in 38,000 red cell units is transfused to the wrong patient. When the wrong unit of blood is given, it is ABO-incompatible 1 in 3 times. Two thirds of these erroneous transfusions are caused by a clerical or management error in identifying the patient, blood sample or blood component and one third are due to an error in the transfusion service. Of these ABO-incompatible transfusions, about 10% are associated with a fatal hemolytic transfusion reaction. Occasionally, a non-ABO antibody may also trigger acute intravascular hemolysis. Very rarely, an antibody from transfused donor plasma may be implicated in an acute hemolytic reaction.

Etiology: The pathophysiology of acute hemolytic reactions involves 3 phases.
- In the first phase, IgM or IgG antibody binds to the transfused red blood cell membranes. If these antibodies are capable of activating complement (C1 to C9), hemolysis occurs.
- In phase 2, the red cells that are not hemolyzed can bind to phagocytic cells through IgG or C3b receptors, stimulating the production of cytokines such as IL-8 and TNF alpha. Bound red cells are destroyed by phagocytosis.
- In phase 3, the systemic effects of anaphylotoxins, C3a and C5a, and cytokines produce the clinical signs and symptoms of an acute hemolytic reaction.

Symptoms: Initial symptoms of hemolysis may include fever, chills, a burning sensation at the IV site, flank pain, anxiety, and tightness in the chest. Clinical signs include tachycardia, fever and hypotension. Anesthetized patients may exhibit only hemoglobinuria, hemoglobinemia or oozing of blood from cut surfaces. Renal failure and DIC may subsequently occur.

Consequences: The morbidity and mortality of hemolytic reactions is proportional to the amount of incompatible blood transfused. Symptoms and signs may occur after transfusion of as little as 1 mL of incompatible blood. Pronounced signs and symptoms are common after 5 to 20 mL. Life-threatening consequences include acute renal failure, shock and DIC. The risk of a fatal reaction is much higher after transfusion of more than 200 mL of incompatible blood.

Lab Data: When a hemolytic reaction is suspected, immediate action must be taken to determine its etiology and minimize its consequences.
- Lavender top tube of blood should be centrifuged and the plasma examined for hemoglobin. A pre-reaction specimen should be used for comparison. Pink or red discoloration in the post-reaction, but not the pre-reaction specimen, may indicate a hemolytic reaction.
- Transfusion Service performs Tier One and Tier Two testing.

The most useful tests to document the occurrence of a hemolytic transfusion reaction are
- Examining the plasma for hemolysis
- A direct antiglobulin test
- Hemoglobin level

If no free hemoglobin is detected in the plasma and the patients' RBCs are not coated with antibody, a hemolytic reaction is highly unlikely. If either test is positive, a hemolytic reaction probably occurred. The hemoglobin or hematocrit should also be checked to see if the expected rise per unit of 1 g/dL for hemoglobin or 3% for hematocrit was achieved. If not, transfused red cells may have been hemolyzed.

A plasma haptoglobin should be performed on both pre and post-transfusion serum specimens. After transfusion of several units of stored blood, the post-transfusion haptoglobin level may be decreased to 50% of the pre-transfusion level, even though the units were compatible. After hemolysis, the pre-transfusion level will be within the reference range of 100 to 150 mg/dL and the post-transfusion level will be zero.

If hemolysis has occurred coagulation tests including PT, aPTT, fibrinogen, platelet count and D-Dimer should be ordered to determine if DIC is occurring. BUN and creatinine should be monitored to assess renal function.

Treatment:
The transfusion should be stopped immediately, but the IV line should be kept open with Normal Saline infusion since hypotension, acute renal failure and shock may occur. Vital signs and urine output should be monitored. Medical consultation may be necessary for management of severe complications.

Prevention: Acute hemolytic reactions are prevented by meticulous attention to patient identification protocols and the introduction of technological advances such as bar coded wristbands. All blood samples drawn for testing must be positively identified. An additional safety measure in the transfusion service is to require that a patient have two blood types on file before ABO specific blood components are issued. Two persons should always verify the identification of the patient and the blood component at the bedside prior to transfusion.

Nonimmune Hemolysis
When symptoms of hemolysis are observed and antibody detection tests are negative, other causes of hemolysis should be investigated including:

- Improper storage or transport of blood (freezing, thawing, overheating, outdating)
- Malfunctioning blood warmer or warming blood by nonapproved methods
- Contact with hypotonic IV solutions in the donor bag or infusion line
- Medications (osmotic or immune hemolysis)
- Large volume infusions of hypotonic solutions
- Older RBCs infused under pressure or with an IV pump
- Mechanical trauma from intraoperative blood collection devices
- Mechanical trauma from extracorporeal circulation machines
- Bacterial contamination of a blood component
- Rare red cell membrane defect or hemoglobinopathy in the donor
- Malfunctioning heart valves
- Vasculitis, TTP or HUS
- Hematoma reabsorption
- Massive trauma or burns
- Infections (clostridia, malaria)
- Congenital & acquired hemolytic anemias in the patient (G6PD, Sickle cell, etc)

The administration of hypotonic solutions with whole blood or red blood cells can cause hemolysis. Solutions containing 5% dextrose are most frequently associated with hemolysis. Besides its osmotic effect, dextrose appears to directly damage red cell membranes, reducing RBC survival. Blood remaining in the administration set tubing should be examined for hemolysis. If the administration set was previously used for infusion of a hypotonic or dextrose solution, hemolysis may be seen in the tubing but not in the blood bag.

Other IV solutions, besides drugs, can also cause adverse effects. Simultaneous administration of hypertonic hyperalimentation or lipid solutions and blood transfusions through multi-lumen catheters has been associated with severe acanthocytosis. The calcium content of Ringer's lactate solution can cause clots to form if it is added to blood component bags or tubing, because of the recalcification of citrated anticoagulated plasma.

Patients with intrinsic red cell defects, such as glucose-6-phosphate dehydrogenase deficiency or sickle cell anemia, may experience intravascular hemolysis unrelated to transfusion. Myoglobinemia, secondary to trauma, may be mistaken for hemolysis.

Symptoms: Hemoglobinuria is present, but other symptoms of acute hemolysis are absent.

Consequences: Adverse effects of nonimmune hemolysis are usually limited.

Lab Data: Hemoglobinuria and hemoglobinemia are observed, but no serological incompatibility is detected. Tier one and tier two testing are completed to rule out an acute hemolytic reaction.

Treatment: Usually no treatment is necessary, but the patient must be monitored closely. The cause of hemolysis needs to be corrected in order to minimize complications.

Prevention: Blood Bank transfusion policies are designed to avoid many situations that contribute to non-immune hemolysis. Careful adherence to policies and patient monitoring will minimize this problem.

Transfusion Related Acute Lung Injury (TRALI)
Transfusion-related acute lung injury (TRALI) is a clinical syndrome that presents as acute hypoxemia and noncardiogenic pulmonary edema within 6 hours after completion of a transfusion of one or more plasma containing blood components, which is not temporally related to another cause of acute lung injury such as pneumonia, gastric aspiration, toxic inhalation, sepsis, shock, and cardio-pulmonary bypass. Today, TRALI is the most frequent cause of transfusion-related death reported to the FDA.

Etiology: Substantial circumstantial evidence indicates that the majority of cases of TRALI are caused by transfusion of plasma containing leukocyte antibodies. Many recipients who develop TRALI have received a donor unit containing antibodies directed against an antigen present on their leukocytes. Such antibodies may be directed against HLA Class I or Class II antigens or non-HLA neutrophil antigens (HNA). The highest frequency of leukocyte antibodies is found in female donors who have previously been pregnant. Overall, about 15 to 20% of female donors have HLA antibodies compared to <1% of male donors.

Several years ago, investigators from the United Kingdom (UK) Serious Hazards of Transfusion (SHOT) system determined that the rate of TRALI occurrence was 5 to 7-fold greater for blood components that contained high volumes of plasma such as FFP and platelets than for packed red blood cells. This data also showed that the majority of TRALI cases involved a leukocyte antibody-positive female donor. On the basis of the SHOT analysis, the UK adopted a policy to minimize the transfusion of FFP and platelets from female donors. Since the implementation of this policy in October 2003, the number of TRALI cases has decreased from 20 per year to 3.

Recently, the American Red Cross analyzed cases of fatal TRALI reported between 2003 and 2005. Retrospective review of fatalities revealed 38 cases of probable TRALI, the majority of which (24 of 38) followed plasma transfusion. A female leukocyte antibody-positive donor was involved in 75% of cases involving plasma and in 60% of cases involving apheresis platelets.

Patients at greatest risk of developing TRALI include those who have undergone recent surgery, induction chemotherapy, cardiopulmonary bypass, massive transfusion, plasma exchange for TTP, or have recently aspirated gastric contents or developed sepsis.

All blood components containing plasma have been implicated in TRALI cases, but the greatest risk is associated with those components containing the largest volume of plasma such as plasma, platelets and cryoprecipitate.

Symptoms: The NHLBI Working Group on TRALI has officially defined this syndrome as a new episode of acute lung injury (ALI) that occurs during or within 6 hours after completion of a transfusion of one or more plasma containing blood components, which is not temporally related to another cause of ALI. Other causes of ALI include:

Direct Lung Injury	Indirect Lung Injury
Aspiration of gastric contents	Sepsis
Pneumonia	Shock
Toxic Inhalation	Multiple trauma
Lung contusion	Burn injury
Near drowning	Acute pancreatitis
	Cardiopulmonary bypass
	Drug overdose

The recommended clinical criteria for diagnosis of TRALI include:
- Acute onset (most cases occur within 1-2 hours of transfusion)
- Hypoxemia
    - PaO2/FiO2<300
    - Oxygen saturation <90% on room air measured by pulse oximetery
- Bilateral pulmonary infiltrates on frontal chest x-ray
- No evidence of circulatory overload

The most frequently observed findings in TRALI cases include dyspnea, tachypnea, cyanosis, fever, tachycardia, hypotension or hypertension, froth in endotracheal tube, and mechanical ventilation required to support oxygenation. TRALI in thrombocytopenic stem cell transplant patients with recovering neutrophils may be diagnosed as diffuse alveolar hemorrhage.

Consequences: Between 6 and 10% of cases are fatal. TRALI must be recognized promptly and treated appropriately. The patient's physician should be notified immediately.

Prevention
AABB has recommended that all blood collecting facilities take steps to minimize the preparation of high plasma-volume components from donors known to be at increased risk of leukocyte alloimmunization. Accordingly, blood centers have begun supplying FFP from only male donors. They also must develop a plan to reduce the risk from apheresis platelets from male donors by March 2008 and implement it by November 2008. This plan may include collecting platelet pheresis from male donors only or male donors and nulliparous female donors. Alternatively, donors may be tested for HLA and granulocyte antibodies.

The blood center supplying a unit implicated in a TRALI case should be notified so that the donor plasma can be tested for leukocyte antibody. Donors testing positive will be permanently deferred from future donations. Patients who develop TRALI are unlikely to have another reaction because it is most often donor specific.

Lab Data: Investigation of a suspected TRALI case
1. Adverse reaction is reported to hospital Transfusion Service
2. Medical Director of Transfusion Service determines if the adverse reaction meets the criteria for diagnosis of TRALI. Other adverse reactions to transfusion may produce similar signs and symptoms. The differential diagnosis includes:
   - Transfusion associated circulatory overload (TACO)
   - Severe allergic or anaphylactic reactions
   - Bacterial contamination
   - Acute hemolytic reaction, usually secondary to ABO incompatibility
   - Acute event unrelated to transfusion; myocardial infarction, pulmonary embolism, sepsis, pneumonia
3. Transfusion service will retrieve a sample of blood from the patient as close as possible to the onset of TRALI.
4. Hospital transfusion service notifies the blood center. Testing for antibodies to HLA class I & II and human neutrophil antigens (HNA) should be confined to donors whose components were transfused within 6 hours preceding the onset of TRALI. The most likely candidates include:
   a. Donors whose components were administered closest to TRALI onset
   b. Donors of plasma>platelets>cryoprecipitate>red blood cells
   c. Donors who are multiparous females>other females>male donors
5. If antibody is detected, its specificity for the recipients' WBC antigens can be determined by either determining the HLA and HNA type of the recipient or performing a crossmatch of donor serum with recipient's WBCs.
6. A donor that is implicated in TRALI will be permanently deferred from future donation.
7. When ALI is temporally related to both transfusion and at least one of these other risk factors, the reaction should be classified as possible TRALI.
8. Fatal cases of TRALI must be reported to FDA and nonfatal cases to MedWatch.
9. Patients with TRALI usually have a normal BNP, which may be helpful in distinguishing TRALI from TACO.

TRALI cases associated with antibody in the recipient reacting with donor WBCs are rare and usually occur after transfusion of nonleukocyte reduced units. Testing would not influence donor management.

Treatment: The transfusion should be stopped. Symptomatic support includes oxygen administration and possibly intubation with mechanical ventilation. Diuretics are not useful in treatment of TRALI because the underlying pathology involves microvascular injury, rather than fluid overload. Corticosteroids are often used empirically but their effectiveness has not been proven.

Prevention: If antibodies are present, the blood center should be notified so that the donor will be permanently deferred from future donations. Patients who develop TRALI are unlikely to have another reaction because it is most often donor specific.

Circulatory Overload

Circulatory overload may occur when excessive volumes of blood or components are administered too quickly. This complication occurs most frequently in patients with severe chronic anemia because they have an expanded blood volume. Infants, elderly adults, and patients with heart or kidney disease are also more prone to develop circulatory overload. When too much blood is transfused too quickly, these patients cannot handle the volume increase and consequently develop heart failure and acute pulmonary edema.

Symptoms: Symptoms include dyspnea, orthopnea, wheezing, tightness in the chest, dry cough, headache, cyanosis, tachypnea, and rapid increase in blood pressure. Peripheral and pulmonary edema may also develop.

Consequences: Usually not serious if intervening steps are taken. Potentially life-threatening if not promptly recognized.

Lab Data: No evidence of serological incompatibility.

Treatment: At the first indication, the patient is placed in a sitting position and the transfusion is stopped. If the symptoms progress, oxygen support and IV administration of a rapid acting diuretic may be necessary. If symptoms are severe and urgent, a therapeutic phlebotomy of 200 to 400 mL may be warranted.

Prevention: Prevention includes avoiding unnecessary fluids, using concentrated components and not transfusing more than 2 units per day. For very unstable patients, it may be necessary to split a unit into two aliqouts and transfuse one half of a unit very slowly at a flow rate not exceeding 1 mL/kg of body weight per hour. Diuretics can also be given prior to transfusion.

Bacterial Contamination

Blood components are sterile. However, if bacteria are introduced into donor units during collection, processing, or pooling, they may cause sepsis or life-threatening endotoxic shock. Recent data has demonstrated that approximately 1 in 5000 apheresis platelets is contaminated with bacteria and 1 in 70,000 to 1 in 118,000 units is associated with a septic transfusion reaction. The reported rate of fatal transfusion reactions due to bacterial sepsis has been less than 1 in a million.

Etiology: Contamination of the donor unit at the time of collection is probably the most common cause of contamination. A small core of skin containing bacteria may enter the phlebotomy needle during skin puncture. Needles, anticoagulant-preservative solution or the plastic blood collection bags and tubing may become contaminated with airborne or waterborne bacteria. A less common source is a donor who has recently recovered from gastroenteritis and is asymptomatic but still bacteremic. Donor bacteremia may also occur during the incubation periods of upper respiratory tract infections and following dental procedures.

Septic reactions are more common after platelet than red blood cell transfusions. Platelets are stored for up to five days at room temperature and provide better growth media for bacteria than do refrigerated red blood cells. The risk of bacterial contamination is less for single donor apheresis platelets than for pooled random donor platelet concentrates.

Symptoms: Sepsis due to contaminated blood components should be suspected if a patient develops high fever, rigors, and profound hypotension shortly after starting a transfusion. Shock, hemolysis, renal failure, and disseminated intravascular coagulation are also frequently present.

Consequences: Transfusion of a bacterially contaminated blood component is potentially fatal. It must be recognized and treated immediately.

Lab data: The transfusion should be stopped immediately and the bag, tubing and other fluids being administered should be returned to the transfusion service for immediate investigation. The bag should be inspected for discoloration, clots or hemolysis. A Gram stain and blood culture should be performed on an aliquot of blood from the bag and from the recipient. The Gram stain may be negative in one third of cases even though contamination is present.

Most Commonly Isolated Bacterial Contaminants

Platelets	Red Cells
Staphylococcus aureus	Yersinia enterocolitica
Klebsiella	Serratia species
Seratia	Pseudomonas species
Staphylococcus epidermidis	
Streptococcus viridans	
Salmonella	
Psuedomonas	
Enterobacter	
E. coli	
Bacillus	
Proteus mirabilis	

Before starting antibiotic therapy, a blood culture should be obtained from the patient. Isolation of the same organism from the blood bag and the patient establishes the diagnosis of bacterial contamination with a high degree of certainty. If the patient is receiving antibiotics at the time of transfusion, blood cultures from the patient may be negative for the organism in question.

Treatment: The patient's physician should be notified immediately. If the patient is not already being treated with IV antibiotics, they should be started as quickly as possible.

Prevention: Each apheresis platelet unit is cultured from the first day after collection until it outdates. If bacterial growth is detected in a unit, a blood center immediately notifies the hospital transfusion service. The hospital transfusion service then takes the following actions:

- If the unit has not been transfused, it is immediately quarantined and returned to the blood center.
- If the unit has already been transfused to an inpatient, the nursing unit is immediately notified.
- If the unit has already been transfused to an outpatient, the ordering physician is immediately contacted.

All policies involving collection, handling, and storage of blood components must be carefully followed. All blood components should be inspected prior to transfusion for any abnormal color, opacity, hemolysis or clots. Suspect units should not be issued for transfusion. The infusion set should be primed and the blood bag spiked using aseptic technique. Transfusions should be begun as soon as the units are available and the transfusion completed within 4 hours to prevent possible bacterial proliferation. If the transfusion cannot be started within 30 minutes the unit should be promptly returned to the Blood Bank for proper storage. If a unit is contaminated, all other blood components from that donation should be immediately recalled.

LATE ONSET REACTIONS

Hemolytic Transfusion Reaction

Etiology: Delayed hemolytic reactions occur in patients who have undetectable levels of antibody when pretransfusion testing is performed, so that seemingly compatible units of red blood cells are transfused. Exposure to antigen positive red blood cells provokes an anamnestic response and increased synthesis of the corresponding antibody. After several days, the antibody titer becomes high enough to hemolyze transfused red cells.

Symptoms: In most cases, delayed hemolytic reactions are asymptomatic and the only noticeable sign is a more rapid fall in the post-transfusion hemoglobin level than is clinically expected. Occasionally a patient experiences a flu-like illness. Fever is the most common symptom, followed by jaundice. In rare instances, hemolysis may be brisk (especially when Kidd antibodies are implicated) resulting in fever, hemoglobinemia and hemoglobinuria.

Consequences: Generally, delayed hemolytic reactions do not result in serious adverse sequelae. Occasionally, the decrease in a patient's hemoglobin associated with a delayed hemolytic transfusion reaction may be misdiagnosed as internal bleeding.

Lab Data: Delayed hemolytic transfusion reactions are most often detected by the blood bank when laboratory tests reveal a positive direct antiglobulin test and/or an indirect antiglobulin test. Other lab findings include decreasing hemoglobin or hematocrit, increasing indirect bilirubin, and positive antibody screen posttransfusion.

Treatment: Treatment is rarely necessary. Urine output and renal function should be monitored. Transfusion of antigen negative blood may be necessary for treatment of anemia.

Prevention: It is critical that the responsible antibody is identified and all additional units are negative for the corresponding antigen. When RBC antibodies are identified, physicians should inform their patients and counsel them to provide this information when they are hospitalized elsewhere. Carrying a transfusion alert card is recommended. Physicians whose patients tell them about previously identified antibodies should immediately notify the Transfusion Service.

Transfusion Associated Graft Versus Host Disease

Etiology: Transfusion associated graft versus host disease (TA-GVHD) occurs when viable donor T lymphocytes engraft and multiply in a recipient incapable of eliminating them. Donor T cells initiate a cell mediated immune response directed at recipient tissue antigens. The recipient's inability to eliminate these donor lymphocytes may result from severe immunodeficiency or an inability to immunologically recognize the transfused cells as foreign. An example of the former is a bone marrow transplant recipient whose immune system has been ablated by high dose chemotherapy. The latter situation occurs in immunocompetent patients who receive directed donations of red cells from first degree relatives or HLA matched platelets. It seems to occur when the donor is homozygous for one of the recipient's HLA haplotypes. For example, if a donor is homozygous for an HLA haplotype (e.g. HLA A2 A2, B7, B7) and a recipient is heterozygous (HLA A2, A19, B7, B57) the recipient would not recognize donor lymphocytes as foreign, but donor lymphocytes would recognize recipient lymphocytes as foreign. The relative risk of TA-GVHD varies with the relationship of donor and recipient.

Relative Risk of TA-GVHD

Donor Relationship	Relative Risk of TA-GVHD
Parent/Child	7.2
Second Degree Relative	4.1
Sibling	3.9
First Cousin	2.6
Second Cousin	1.4
Unrelated	1.0

Symptoms: Patients with TA-GVHD display the classic signs of fever, erythematous maculopapular skin rash, diarrhea, hepatomegaly, elevation of liver enzymes, lymphadenopathy and severe pancytopenia. The onset of symptoms may occur from 2 to 30 days after transfusion.

Comparison of Transfusion & Transplantation GVHD

	TA-GVHD	BMT-GVHD
Onset	2 to 30 days	35 to 70 days
Pancytopenia	Yes	No
Duration	<54 days	Longer
Fatality rate	90%	<5%

Consequences: The response to therapy is poor and mortality is 90%. Most patients die from severe pancytopenia and infection.

Prevention: TA-GVHD can be prevented by gamma irradiation (2500 cGy per unit for 1 to 5 minutes) of cellular blood components to inactivate lymphocytes. Leukocyte reduction by filtration does not remove sufficient numbers of lymphocytes to prevent graft versus host disease.

Treatment: No treatment has proven to be effective.

Iron Accumulation
Etiology: Each unit of red blood cells contains about 250 mg of iron complexed with hemoglobin. Transfusion hemosiderosis may become apparent after about 100 units of blood. Organ damage may already be advanced at the time of diagnosis. Organ toxicity begins when reticuloendothelial sites of iron storage become saturated and iron becomes deposited in other cells. Iron causes oxidative damage to liver, heart and endocrine glands.

Consequences: The most serious complication is cardiotoxicity, which may lead to arrhythmias, congestive heart failure and death. Hepatic injury, diabetes mellitus and adrenal insufficiency may also occur.

Lab Data: Serial ferritin monitoring is helpful in assessing total body iron burden.

Treatment: Treatment with iron chelation agents, such as parenteral deferoxamine, should be initiated early in the course of chronic transfusion therapy. Long term maintenance of serum ferritin below 300 ng/mL is associated with improved survival.

Prevention: The best way to prevent iron overload is to limit the number of transfusions as much as possible.

Transfusion Transmitted Diseases
Transfusion transmitted infectious diseases usually share the following properties;

- Long period of subclinical infection
- Lengthy viremic phase or carrier state
- Survivability in stored blood components

The following viruses are known to be transmitted by transfusion.

Viruses Transmitted by Transfusion

Plasma Associated	Cell Associated
Hepatitis A	Cytomegalovirus
Hepatitis B	Epstein Barr Virus
Hepatitis C	HTLV-1
HIV-1	HTLV-2
HIV-2	HIV-1
West Nile	HIV-2
	Parvovirus B19

Hepatitis
Before the late 1970's, the risk of transmitting hepatitis by transfusion was very high because of blood collection from prisoners and paid donors and the lack of sensitive serological tests. Between 1965 and 1972, approximately 1 in 60 units of blood transmitted hepatitis. The change to an all-volunteer blood supply and the introduction of a third generation test for HBsAg in the mid 1970's led to a marked reduction in transfusion transmitted hepatitis B infection. The risk decreased even further with the implementation of ALT and anti-HBc tests in 1987 and 1988 as surrogate markers for hepatitis C. Today the risk of transmitting hepatitis B is only 1 case per 205,0000 units and it accounts for only 10% of post-transfusion hepatitis cases. Further reduction may occur, as hepatitis B vaccination becomes more widespread and nucleic acid testing is adopted.

In the late 1970's, approximately 10% of patients who were transfused with multiple units of red cells became infected with hepatitis C. The introduction of more stringent donor eligibility criteria and both serological and nucleic acid tests hepatitis C virus antibody and RNA has reduced the risk of transmission to about 1 infection per 2,000,000 units transfused.

The natural history of transfusion acquired HCV is similar to that of HCV acquired through other modes of transmission. Approximately 50% of patients will develop chronic elevations of liver enzymes and 10% of these will develop cirrhosis.

HIV-1
The risk of transmitting HIV-1 by transfusion has almost been completely eliminated over the past 25 years. The risk has decreased from 1 case per 100 transfused units in 1983 to 1 case per 2 million today. The risk declined dramatically with the identification and deferral of donors with high-risk behavior in 1983 and the introduction of HIV-1 antibody testing in 1985. In late 1995, blood banks began to test donors for p24 antigen to identify donors in the window period of an early infection who did not have detectable antibody. P24 antigen testing decreased the window period from 22 to 16 days. In late 1999, blood banks introduced nucleic acid testing for HIV-1 RNA to further reduce the possibility that a unit collected during the window period might be transfused. The window period is now estimated to be 11 days.

HIV-2
HIV-2 also causes AIDS and can be transmitted by blood. The FDA licensed the first combination test kit for detecting antibodies to HIV-1 and HIV-2 on September 25, 1992. All blood

centers were required to implement this combination test by June 1993. Very few cases of HIV-2 have been detected in the United States. The risk of transmitting HIV-2 by blood transfusion is very small.

HTLV

In 1988, the first generation HTLV-1 antibody test was licensed in the U.S. to screen blood donors for human T cell lymphotropic virus type 1 (HTLV-1), which is a retrovirus that has been associated with adult T cell leukemia (ATCL) and a neurological syndrome, HTLV-1 associated myelopathy (HAM). Cellular blood products including red blood cells, platelets and granulocytes can transmit HTLV-1. Plasma components such as FFP and cryoprecipitate do not. Storage of cellular components for more than 14 days appears to decrease infectivity. Between 20 and 60% of recipients who received HTLV-1 positive units prior to the introduction of testing, have seroconverted.

Another related virus, HTLV-2, was originally isolated from patients with hairy cell leukemia. It is transmitted by blood and sexual intercourse. Most males in the United States with HTLV-2 infection have a history of drug abuse, while most infected females have a history of sexual contact with a known IV drug user. Because this virus is closely related to HTLV-1, the HTLV-1 antibody test detects the majority of HTLV-2 positive blood donors. A separate test that could specifically identify HTLV-2 antibody was implemented in 1992.

Disease associations arising from HTLV-1 or HTLV-II infection are much less frequent than HIV. It has been estimated that 4% of individuals infected with HTLV-1 at birth may progress to ATCL during their lifetime, usually after an incubation period of at least 20 to 30 years. HAM has been estimated to occur in 0.25% of persons infected with HTLV-1 after an incubation period of months to years. A similar neurological syndrome has been documented as a result of HTLV-II infection. However, there is no evidence linking HTLV-II infection with ATCL.

CMV

Cytomegalovirus (CMV) is present within the leukocytes of at least 60% of adult blood donors. However, only 1% of seropositive units is infectious. Only cellular blood components transmit CMV infection. Clinical disease is rare in immunocompetent recipients presumably because they have protective CMV antibody levels. Adverse effects are usually limited to heterophile negative mononucleosis syndromes or mild hepatitis. Transfusion transmitted CMV infections can cause serious illness in CMV negative patients who are immunocompromised, such as premature infants (<1250 g), bone marrow and solid organ transplant recipients and CMV negative AIDS patients. Clinical manifestations include hepatitis, retinitis, pneumonitis, encephalitis and GI tract disease. Intrauterine infection may cause jaundice, thrombocytopenia, cerebral infarction and mental retardation.

The risk of transfusion associated CMV infection may be essentially eliminated by transfusing blood components that are leukocyte reduced (<5 x 106 WBCs) or are CMV seronegative.

West Nile Virus

WNV is a mosquito-borne virus that is associated with meningitis and encephalitis. It was first recognized as a transfusion transmitted agent in 2002. Red blood cells, platelets, and fresh frozen plasma have been implicated in transfusion-transmitted disease.

A potential donor with a medical diagnosis of West Nile virus or suspected of having a WNV infection is deferred for 120 days after diagnosis or onset of illness, whichever occurred later. Nucleic acid tests (NAT) for WNV in donated blood were implemented on July 1, 2003.

Variant Creutzfeldt-Jakob disease

Bovine spongiform encephalopathy (BSE), also known as mad cow disease, is a transmissible spongiform encephalopathy that is responsible for the human neurodegenerative disorder known as variant Creutzfeldt-Jakob disease (vCJD). BSE first appeared in cattle in the United Kingdom (UK) in 1986. The origin of BSE is thought to be cattle feed containing meat & bone meal supplements contaminated by scrapie infected sheep carcasses. Similarly, vCJD was transmitted to humans through consumption of beef products contaminated by infected neural tissue, such as hot dogs, sausages, lunchmeat, meat pies and various canned meat goods. BSE infections in the UK have decreased substantially since 1992 due to slaughter of infected animals and changes in animal feed production. BSE has not occurred in the US or other countries that do not import live cattle, beef products, or livestock nutritional supplements from the UK. In December 2003, the United Kingdom Health Secretary reported the world's first possible case of variant Creutzfeldt Jakob disease (vCJD) by transfusion of red blood cells. The blood donor, who was free of symptoms at the time of donation, donated in March 1996.

The incubation period of vCJD is not known. If large numbers of infected persons are silently incubating the disease, human to human iatrogenic spread may be possible .The disease could unknowingly be spread during invasive medical and surgical procedures and donation of organs, tissues and blood.

No sensitive screening tests currently exist. The FDA has taken several measures to prevent future transmission. In 1999, FDA mandated that blood centers must defer donors who:

- Spent greater than 3 months in the United Kingdom from 1980 through 1996
- Lived on a military base in Europe between 1980 and 1996
- Were transfused in the United Kingdom since 1980
- Lived more than 5 years in Europe
- Been injected with bovine insulin since 1980
- Have a family history of CJD
- Been a recipient of a dura mater graft or human pituitary derived growth hormone.

Since 1998, the UK has used only leukocyte reduced blood because experts on prion diseases consider white blood cells to be a potential source of infection.

Trypanosoma cruzi

Chaga's disease is caused by the parasite, *Trypanosoma cruzi*. As many as 11 million persons in Mexico and in Central and South America carry the parasite and serve as a potential source of transfusion transmitted disease. The risk of *T. cruzi* transmission in the United States is increasing because of immigration of infected individuals from endemic countries. Estimates of the incidence of seropositive donors in the United States have ranged from 1 in 5400 to 1 in 25,000 donors.

Transfusion of red blood cells and platelets from infected donors carries the highest risk of transmission, approximately 38%. The risk of transmission from plasma components is considerably lower because *T. cruzi* is killed by freezing. The lifetime risk of severe heart or intestinal problems in infected individuals averages about 30% and usually occurs many years after the initial infection.

Testing of donors for antibodies to *Trypanosoma cruzi* was introduced in 2007, since persons with acute infections remain asymptomatic for long periods of time and Typanosoma cruzi can survive for several weeks in refrigerated blood. FDA requires hospitals to participate in a Look-back program which involves identification of all recipients of previously transfused blood components from confirmed positive donors. Individuals with a history of Chagas disease are permanently deferred from donating blood.

CHAPTER 8:
Transfusion Therapy

RED BLOOD CELLS

Red blood cells (RBCs) are the cells that remain following separation of plasma from whole blood at any time during storage. RBCs preserved with Adsol contain approximately 30 to 40 mL of CPD plasma, 100 mL of Adsol solution, and 150 – 230 mL of red cells and have a shelf life of 42 days. The hematocrit is 55 to 80%. RBCs produced without Adsol contain approximately 70 mL of CPDA1 plasma, have a hematocrit of 70 to 80% and a shelf life of 35 days.

Treatment of Acute Anemia

Transfusion of RBCs is indicated to increase oxygen delivery in patients who are actively bleeding and in those who have symptomatic anemia unresponsive to specific therapy. The primary therapy for acute hemorrhage is volume replacement with crystalloid, because the treatment of or prevention of hypovolemic shock is more important than restoration of oxygen carrying capacity. If symptoms persist after volume repletion, red cell transfusion should be considered. Symptoms include syncope, pallor, dyspnea, postural hypotension, tachycardia, angina, transient ischemic attacks, and others noted below. The presence of these symptoms indicates that the patient was unable to compensate for the reduced oxygen carrying capacity. The normal compensatory mechanisms include increased cardiac output, peripheral vasoconstriction and increased oxygen extraction by peripheral tissues. These symptoms can be used to estimate the percentage of blood loss.

Signs & Symptoms of Acute Blood Loss

Blood Loss (mL)	% Blood Volume	Signs & Symptoms
500	8	none
1000 - 1500	16 - 20	tachycardia (110-120), exercise tachypnea, postural hypotension
1500 - 2000	20 - 30	tachycardia at rest (120), hypotension (90 mm systolic), sweating, air hunger, anxiety, restlessness
2000	40	severe hypotension (60 mm systolic)
>2000	50	severe hypotension, pale, cold, ashen, drowsy or unconscious

The loss of 500 mL of blood within 5 minutes is well tolerated by the average adult blood donor. Therefore, it is usually not necessary to transfuse patients with a single unit of RBCs since the recipient probably needs the blood no more than the donor. Patients who have suddenly lost more than 20 to 30% of their blood volume are more critical and develop symptoms in spite of compensatory mechanisms such as peripheral vasoconstriction and fluid shift from the extravascular to the intravascular space. Hemodilution begins almost immediately after the onset of hemorrhage and continues up to 72 h after cessation of bleeding. Although this influx of fluid does not improve oxygen carrying capacity, it does help to maintain blood volume and stabilize circulation. In this situation, transfusion of a single unit of RBCs along with crystalloid solutions is justifiable since the patient has lost the equivalent of three units of blood. Adult patients in hemorrhagic shock have usually lost 35 to 40% of their blood volume, or approximately 2 liters.

Blood volume should be immediately replaced with crystalloid solutions such as lactated Ringer's solution or normal saline. The early administration of fluids allows sufficient time for ABO typing of the recipient, which takes only a few minutes. In this way, ABO type specific blood can be given instead of empirically giving O negative blood, which often is in short supply.

Numerous publications have debated the risks and benefits of using hemoglobin levels between 6 and 10 g/dL as a transfusion trigger for patients with acute blood loss. Generally, isovolemic patients with a hemoglobin <7 g/dL may require transfusion, while most patients with a hemoglobin >9 g/dL will not.

The Transfusion Requirements in Critical Care Trial (TRICC) was a multi-center prospective randomized controlled clinical trial conducted in Canada in 1999, which compared the clinical outcomes in intensive care patients randomized to a restrictive versus a liberal transfusion strategy (NEJM 1999; 340: 409-17). Patients in the restrictive cohort were transfused when their hemoglobin concentration fell below 7 g/dL and their hemoglobin was maintained between 7–9 g/dL, while patients in the liberal transfusion group were transfused when their hemoglobin concentration fell below 10 g/dL and their hemoglobin was maintained between 10–12 g/dL.

TRICC Trial Outcomes

Outcomes	Liberal	Restrictive
#Patients	420	418
#RBC units	5.2+/-4.9	2.5+/-3.8
Transfusion avoidance	0%	33%
ICU stay	11.5 days	11.0 days
30 day survival	77%	81%
60 day survival	74%	77%

The TRICC trial demonstrated that a more restrictive transfusion strategy was safe in the ICU patient population and that the liberal use of transfusions increased the risk of death. Multiple other studies have subsequently demonstrated that allogeneic transfusions cause immunomodulation leading to increased ICU and hospital length of stay as well as nosocomial infections and mortality.

Transfusion medicine has evolved over the last few years. Because allogeneic transfusions are a potential risk for patients, physicians should attempt to limit transfusions by aggressively preventing anemia in hospitalized patients. The decision to transfuse RBCs should be based on the entire clinical picture and not solely on the hemoglobin level.

Reversible causes of chronic anemia such as vitamin B12, folate, and iron deficiency should be ruled out prior to transfusion. Erythropoietin sensitive anemia such as anemia of chronic renal insufficiency and the anemia associated with zidovudine (AZT) treatment of HIV patients should also be ruled out. Red cell transfusions may be required to alleviate the symptoms of anemia or to reduce morbidity associated with a patient's underlying disease. Symptoms in normovolemic patients that may indicate the need for transfusion include dyspnea, syncope, transient ischemic attacks, postural hypotension, tachycardia, tachypnea, and angina.

Chronic anemia patients undergo compensatory changes that acclimate them to lower hemoglobin levels. A point of fundamental importance is that blood volume is decreased only slightly in patients with chronic anemia due to compensatory increases in plasma volume. Thus, transfusion of chronically anemic patients may cause hypervolemia which has the potential for precipitating cardiac decompensation, particularly in elderly patients or in patients with known heart failure.

Physicians must not be overly aggressive in the transfusion of patients with severe anemia. Transfusion will improve functional status in symptomatic patients up to a hemoglobin level of 10 g/dL. Transfusions beyond this level provide no further improvement in functional status in most patients. This is especially true for patients with impaired cardiac output because their inability to compensate for increased blood viscosity can actually decrease tissue oxygenation. The major exception is patients with severe chronic obstructive pulmonary disease (COPD) who may still be symptomatic at hemoglobin levels of 10 g/dL and require a hemoglobin level between 10 and 12g/dL to alleviate symptoms. Patients taking medications, such as beta-blockers, may not be able to mount an adequate sympathetic response to blood loss. Transfusion to a hemoglobin level of 10 g/dL may be necessary to relieve symptoms.

Transfusion in the Setting of Angina
Angina may be indicative of an impending myocardial infarction. Indications for transfusion of patients with myocardial infarction are unclear. Transfusion may improve myocardial oxygen delivery, but may also increase myocardial oxygen consumption secondary to increased blood volume and blood viscosity. The decision to transfuse should be based on critical patient evaluation and internal hemodynamic pressure monitoring. Hemoglobin of 8 g/dL is usually tolerable in surgical patients without risk factors for ischemia, while hemoglobin of 10 g/dL may be better for patients with increased risk. Perioperative myocardial infarction is more likely when the hemoglobin is <9 g/dL, especially if the patient has tachycardia.

Perioperative Transfusion
Red cell transfusion has often been used empirically prior to general anesthesia when the hemoglobin is less than 9 or 10 g/dL. There are no data that strongly support this practice. Rather than use a formula approach, proper preoperative assessment should correlate the adequacy of the hemoglobin level with the cause and duration of the anemia, the patient's cardiac and pulmonary status and the type and probable duration of the surgery. The key to tolerance of anemia is the maintenance of normovolemia and compensatory mechanisms that increase cardiac output and improve oxygen transport. Each patient should be evaluated based upon the anticipated ability of his/ her cardiovascular system to compensate.

Hemodynamic instability may also occur during acute blood loss, usually after loss of 15% or more of blood volume. Accordingly, red cell transfusion is indicated if acute blood loss causes the blood pressure to drop by 20% or to a level of <100 mm Hg, or if the pulse increases to >100/min. The transfusion of colloid and/or crystalloid solutions is also necessary in bleeding patients to maintain adequate blood volume. As long as normovolemia is maintained with colloid and/or crystalloid solutions and the patient's hemoglobin level is adequate, it is not necessary to replace all losses of red cells. Fresh frozen plasma should not be used for volume replacement since this incurs the unnecessary risk of infectious disease transmission.

Postoperative hemoglobin in the range of 8-9 g/dL appears to be safe for patients free of cardiovascular disease, and justification should be provided if blood is transfused other than to replace losses at this level. On the other hand, compensation for acute anemia requires increased cardiovascular performance. Moderate hemodilution (below a hemoglobin of 8-10 g/dL) does affect cardiac workload, and its risks should be weighed carefully in patients with extensive cardiovascular disease .

Each unit increases an adult's (70kg) hemoglobin 1g/dL and hematocrit 3%. Follow up measurement of the recipient's hemoglobin and/or hematocrit can be performed between 15 minutes and 24 hours post-transfusion. The optimal time interval for assessment is 15 minutes. Hemoglobin levels obtained at 24 hours post-transfusion are 10% higher than values obtained after 15 minutes.

PLATELET CONCENTRATES

Platelets for transfusion can be prepared either by separation of platelet concentrates from whole blood or by apheresis from single donors. Comparative studies have shown that post-transfusion increment, platelet survival and hemostatic effect are similar with either product.

Random Donor Platelets
Platelets prepared from whole blood are often referred to as random donor platelet concentrates. Platelet rich plasma is separated from red blood cells by centrifugation at a low G force within 4 hours after donation. Platelet rich plasma is then centrifuged at higher G force and most of the platelet poor plasma supernatant is removed. The remaining platelet concentrate contains between 5.5 and 8.5 X 10^{10} platelets suspended in about 50 mL of plasma. This is approximately 70% of the platelets in the original unit of whole blood.

Platelets are stored at room temperature using continuous gentle horizontal agitation in plastic bags designed to optimize oxygen and carbon dioxide exchange. Platelets can be preserved for 5 days under these conditions. Platelet concentrates are pooled immediately prior to transfusion and can then be stored for 4 hours.

One drawback of random donor platelets is that the concentrates contain 10^8 to 10^9 white blood cells or approximately 50% of the leukocytes from the original unit of whole blood. Random donor platelets should be transfused through a bedside leukocyte reduction filter.

Random donor platelet concentrates may contain up to 0.5 mL of red cells. Transfusion of as little as 0.03 mL of RBCs can stimulate anti-D synthesis. Different studies have demonstrated that 8 to 19% of Rh negative cancer patients form anti-D antibody if transfused with Rh positive platelet concentrates. Rh negative units should be used for Rh negative female children and women of childbearing age. If this is not possible then one vial of Rh immune globulin may be given before or immediately after transfusion with Rh positive platelets. Because these patients are thrombocytopenic, it is preferable to administer anti-D intravenously. A dose of 25 ug (125 IU) will protect against 1 mL of RBCs.

Single Donor Platelets
Apheresis platelets are usually called single donor platelets because they are collected from a single donor with an automated cell separator. Donors usually have an IV line in each arm. Blood pumped from one arm passes through a blood cell separator centrifugation system that collects platelets and returns plasma and red cells to the donor's other arm. Between 4000 and 5000 mL of blood are processed over 1.5 to 2 hours. A single donor platelet concentrate contains a minimum of 3.0 X 10^{11} platelets suspended in approximately 200 mL of plasma, which is the equivalent of 6 to 8 random donor platelet concentrates. They can be stored up to 5 days under the same conditions as random donor platelet concentrates. Five day old apheresis platelets produce the same posttransfusion platelet increment as one day old units.

Single donor apheresis platelets contain fewer than 5×10^6 white blood cells and are considered to be leukocyte reduced. Additional leukocyte reduction filtration is not necessary. Rh negative patients do not need Rh immune globulin after transfusion of Rh positive apheresis platelets because they contain so few red blood cells (0.001 – 0.007 mL).

Single donor platelets offer several advantages over random donor concentrates including:

- Less inventory and pooling
- Fewer donor exposures & fewer lookback investigations
- Leukocyte reduction during collection eliminates the need for bedside filtration

- Ten fold lower risk of bacterial contamination & 5 fold lower risk of septic transfusion reaction
- Easier platelet crossmatching or HLA matching for refractory patients
- Fewer contaminating red blood cells eliminating need for RhIg

Apheresis platelets have a higher processing fee than random donor platelets, but the cost difference is negligible when pooling and leukocyte reduction filter costs are considered.

Platelet ABO Compatibility

The term "ABO-compatible" is confusing when thinking about blood components other than RBCs. Red Blood Cell units contain cells carrying the ABO antigens of the donor and plasma carrying soluble ABO antigens and anti-A and anti-B antibodies. The recipient also possesses ABO antigens and antibodies, but in much larger amounts. Group O blood components do not express cellular and soluble A and B antigens, but do contain anti-A and anti-B antibodies, often in higher titer and avidity than in group A or B components. Group O (so-called universal donor) RBCs usually can be safely transfused to group A or B patients, because the volume of residual incompatible plasma (30 – 70 mL) is minimal. In contrast, a single donor (apheresis) platelet or a pool of 10 random donor platelet concentrates is suspended in 200 to 600 mL of donor plasma. If these platelets are not ABO identical, large volumes of incompatible plasma will be infused, often on a daily basis for extended periods. Anti-A and anti-B can bind to RBCs and to soluble A and B antigens. In the latter instance, immune complexes are formed that can initiate inflammation, tissue injury, and immune suppression. Thus, unlike RBC transfusions, there really are no ABO compatible platelet transfusions. Platelet transfusions should be classified as either ABO identical or nonidentical.

The most obvious adverse effect of transfusing ABO nonidentical platelets is hemolysis. The risk of an ABO hemolytic reaction is rare after a single transfusion of ABO nonidentical platelets, but increases significantly when large volumes are transfused over a relatively short time period. Hemolysis is unlikely after a single ABO incompatible unit for two reasons. First, transfused plasma is diluted almost 10 fold in the patient's intravascular blood volume . Second, and perhaps most importantly, transfused anti-A and anti-B antibodies are rapidly neutralized by binding to circulating soluble A and B antigens as well as tissue A and B antigens. Transfusion of platelets containing large volumes of ABO incompatible plasma saturates soluble and tissue ABO antigen sites and permits binding of excess anti-A and / or anti-B to red blood cells. When this happens, patients develop a positive direct antiglobulin test (DAT) and possibly hemolysis.

Other serious adverse consequences of transfusing ABO nonidentical platelets have also been reported. Chronically transfused patients with hematologic disease who are transfused with nonidentical ABO platelets achieve lower post-transfusion platelet counts, require almost twice as many platelet transfusions, and develop platelet refractoriness earlier than patients receiving ABO identical platelet transfusions. Transfusion of group A or B platelets to group O recipients results in post-transfusion platelet increments that are 20% less than those obtained with ABO identical platelet transfusions. Decreased platelet survival is due to the binding of recipient anti-A and / or anti-B to the transfused donor platelets. Transfusion of group O platelets to group A or B recipients results in even lower post-transfusion platelet increments, suggesting that incompatible plasma is an even more important risk factor. In this situation, anti-A and anti-B in the transfused plasma forms immune complexes with soluble A and / or B antigens circulating in the recipient's plasma. These complexes circulate for hours to days after incompatible transfusions and can bind to platelets resulting in their activation and premature destruction.

Transfusion of ABO nonidentical platelets to transplant patients can have even more deleterious effects. Patients receiving allogeneic marrow or stem cell transplants and patients receiving chemotherapy for acute leukemia have increased mortality due to multi-organ failure and sepsis if they are transfused with ABO nonidentical platelets. ABO antigens, like HLA antigens, are widely expressed on the endothelium lining of blood vessels. Anti-A and/or anti-B antibodies present in ABO incompatible platelets appear to inflict direct damage to organs by binding to endothelial A and B antigens. The formation of anti-A and/or anti-B immune complexes also suppresses cellular immunity, resulting in a predisposition to infection.

Apheresis platelets are preferred over random donor platelets, because of the lower risks associated with a decreased number of donor exposures. If ABO identical apheresis platelets are not available, it is most important to avoid transfusing substantial amounts of anti-A and/or anti-B to patients expressing those antigens. Therefore, the second best choice is to provide random donor ABO identical platelets with a bedside leukocyte reduction filter. When neither apheresis nor random donor ABO identical platelets are available, the ordering physician should be consulted to see if the transfusion could be delayed until ABO identical platelets become available. If immediate transfusion is necessary, the following list can be consulted for additional choices.

- 1st choice is ABO identical apheresis platelet
- 2nd choice is ABO identical random donor platelets with bedside leukocyte reduction filter
- 3rd choice is to see if transfusion can be delayed until ABO identical platelets become available
- 4th choice is ABO nonidentical apheresis platelet
- 5th choice is ABO nonidentical random donor platelets with bedside leukocyte filter

The Transfusion Service should also refrain from infusing substantial amounts of soluble or cell associated A and/or B antigens to patients with detectable levels of the corresponding antibody. The most common example is the transfusion of Group A or B platelets to a group O recipient. This practice is permissible if a patient is hemorrhaging and has a platelet count below 100,000 and neither group O random nor single donor platelets is available.

Platelet Dosage
The dose of platelets should be individualized. A number of simple guidelines can be used to calculate the appropriate dose.

- A dose of 1 random donor platelet concentrate per 10 kg body weight can be expected to increase the platelet count by 5000/uL in a non-refractory patient.
- One random donor platelet concentrate is expected to increase the platelet count by 5000 to 10,000/uL in a 70 kg patient who is not refractory.
- Generally, a pool of 6 to 8 platelet concentrates or a single apheresis unit is sufficient to correct or prevent bleeding in a normal sized adult weighing up to 90 kg.
- One apheresis product is equivalent to 6 to 8 random donor platelet concentrates and therefore should increase the platelet count by 30,000/uL to 40,000/uL in a 70 kg patient.
- For pediatric patients, 5 mL/kg body weight of a random donor platelet concentrate should increase the platelet count by 5000/uL. A single platelet concentrate contains about 45 to 50 mL and should supply the needs of patients up to 8 kg. If the entire platelet concentrate is not used for a given patient, it is not practical to salvage the remainder of the unit.
- For children >8 kg, a standard dose of 1 unit/10 kg should be used.
- In the absence of increased platelet destruction, platelet transfusion will usually need to be repeated every 3-5 days.
- If increased platelet destruction or consumption is present, daily administration may be required.

Anemia is an important risk factor contributing to an increased risk of bleeding, particularly in thrombocytopenic patients and patients with acquired qualitative platelet defects such as uremia. Maintaining these patients' hematocrits at higher levels contributes to improved hemostasis and decreased bleeding. Hemodynamic studies have demonstrated that at higher hematocrits, red blood cells predominate in the central portion of the bloodstream and push platelets peripherally where they are more readily available to interact with endothelium at sites of injury. For this reason, the laboratory recommends that if a patient is both anemic and thrombocytopenic, red blood cells should be transfused before platelets.

Platelet Transfusion Guidelines
The most common reasons for transfusing platelets are:
- Decreased platelet production
- Increased destruction
- Qualitative platelet defects.

Platelet transfusion is generally reserved for patients with impaired marrow production of platelets and should be avoided whenever possible for patients with increased platelet destruction such as autoimmune or drug induced thrombocytopenia. Platelet transfusions are relatively contraindicated in patients with thrombotic thrombocytopenic purpura because of concerns about the risk of precipitating thrombosis.

A. Decreased platelet production:
1. Prophylaxis against spontaneous hemorrhage when:
   - Platelet counts are <10,000/uL.
   - Platelet counts are <20,000/uL with fever, infection or similar condition
   - Platelet counts are <50,000/uL with headache, continued bleeding from a wound or surgical incision, retinal hemorrhage or confluent petechial hemorrhage
2. Bleeding patient with platelet count <50,000/uL. Bleeding includes microvascular bleeding, epistaxis, hematuria, or suspected or proven internal bleeding.
3. Prohylaxis prior to surgery or invasive procedures with platelet count <50,000/uL. Invasive procedures include central venous catheter insertion, dental extractions, transbronchial biopsy, bronchoscopy, bronchoalveolar lavage, GI endoscopy, liver biopsy and lumbar puncture.

B. Increased platelet destruction or consumption
1. Intraoperative use:
   - Platelet count <50,000/uL and nonmechanical or microvascular bleeding.
   - Platelet count <100,00/uL and neurosurgery, middle ear surgery, or ophthhalmologic surgery
   - Platelet count <100,000/uL and ventricular assist devices, cardiopulmonary bypass, or intra-aortic balloon pump
2. Platelet count<50,000/uL during massive transfusion & continued non-mechanical bleeding
3. Platelet count <50,000/uL and bleeding with hypersplenism, sepsis, or DIC
4. Patients with ITP with life- or organ-threatening bleeding or head trauma may require repeated or continuous platelet infusions in addition to immunosuppressive therapy.
5. TTP and hemolytic uremic syndrome if platelet count <10,000/uL or bleeding
6. Neonatal alloimmune thrombocytopenia – washed maternal or antigen negative platelets.

C. Qualitative platelet defects:

1. Congenital defect only if bleeding.
2. Acquired defect if bleeding.
3. Platelet antagonist reversal if bleeding or emergency surgery
   - Aspirin.
   - Plavix (clopidogrel)
   - Reopro (abciximab)
   - Integrilin (eptifibatide)
   - Aggrastat (tirofiban)

Qualitative platelet defects are most often acquired. Uremia, aspirin and other platelet antagonists most commonly cause acquired platelet defects. Platelet transfusions are of limited value in the treatment of acquired disorders, since transfused platelets are also inactivated. They should be limited to treatment of severe bleeding.

Cryoprecipitate transiently corrects uremic platelet defects. Reversal of a qualitative platelet defect requires 10 units of cryoprecipitate. Improvement in platelet function may not be evident for up to 4 hours and lasts approximately 24 hours. Repeat doses of cryoprecipitate are less beneficial. Dialysis also corrects the uremic qualitative platelet defect. Thus, the use of cryoprecipitate to correct a qualitative platelet defect should be reserved for life-threatening hemorrhage or prior to an invasive procedure.

Patients undergoing percutaneous coronary intervention are commonly treated with platelet glycoprotein IIb/IIIa inhibitors (GpIIb/IIIa) such as Reopro, Integrilin and Aggrastat to prevent thrombosis. The platelet binding characteristics of these medications are summarized in the following table.

Platelet Glycoprotein Inhibitors

Generic Name	Abciximab	Eptifibatide	Tirofiban
Brand Name	Reo Pro	Integrilin	Aggrastat
Structure	Fab Ig	Peptide	Peptide
Half Life	10-30 minutes	2.5 hours	2 hours
Affinity	High	Low	Low

Although abciximab is rapidly cleared from plasma, platelet aggregation may be inhibited for 2 to 36 hours after discontinuation of the infusion. Platelet aggregation returns to normal within 0.5 to 4 hours after discontinuation of eptifibatide or tirofiban. If bleeding occurs, infusion of the GPIIb/IIIa inhibitor should be immediately stopped for 30 to 120 minutes. In the event of serious hemorrhaging or emergent surgery, one or two units of single donor platelets may be necessary.

In less than 1% of treated patients, GPIIb/IIIa inhibitors may cause a precipitous drop in the platelet count below 20,000/uL. The onset may be one hour to a few days after exposure. In this situation, it may be necessary to transfuse several units of single donor platelets or one or two batches of random donor platelets may be necessary.

Selective serotonin reuptake inhibitors, such as fluoxetine, sertraline, paroxetine, and clomipramine, decrease the uptake of serotonin by platelets. Since platelets are unable to synthesize serotonin, these medications lower the intracellular serotonin concentration, inhibit platelet aggregation and increase the risk of abnormal bleeding including menorrhagia, metrorrhagia, upper GI hemorrhage, cerebral hemorrhage, hematuria, hemoptysis, hemarthrosis, and post-op bleeding. Platelet transfusions will probably not be effective in controlling bleeding until after these medications have been discontinued for several half-lives.

Monitoring the Effectiveness Of Platelet Transfusions

- A pre-transfusion platelet count should be obtained within 24 hours of ordering a platelet transfusion.

- A post-transfusion platelet count should be done the morning following a platelet transfusion to document the platelet count increment.

- If two consecutive transfusions yield increments that do not meet the minimum standard for a successful transfusion (see Refractoriness below), the effectiveness of subsequent platelet transfusions should be evaluated by performing a count 10 to 60 minutes after their completion.

- When HLA-matched or crossmatched platelets are provided for refractory patients (see below), a platelet count within one hour prior to transfusion and 10-60 minutes following completion of transfusion is necessary to evaluate their effectiveness.

Most nonimmune causes of platelet destruction have a greater effect on the 24 hour post-transfusion platelet count than the 10-60 minutes count. Patients with severe infection or DIC can have a relatively normal immediate post-transfusion platelet count, but a low 24 hour platelet count. Massive splenomegaly, shock and massive transfusion are exceptions to this observation. In contrast, patients with platelet antibody have both markedly shortened 10-60 minute and 24 hour post-transfusion platelet counts. Thus, it is usually possible to distinguish alloimmunization (refractoriness) from other complicating medical factors by measurement of platelet counts immediately after transfusion.

Most platelet transfusions are given prophylactically. This means that platelets are transfused to a patient who has thrombocytopenia, but is not bleeding. In stable patients without other factors that increase the risk of bleeding, the goal is to continuously maintain the platelet count above 10 to 20,000/uL. The immediate posttransfusion platelet count should be >20,000/uL and the platelet count obtained 24 hours later should still be >10,000/uL.

In more unstable patients with other risk factors for bleeding (e.g. medications, liver disease, renal failure, prolonged PT &/or PTT, sepsis, DIC), it is more desirable for the immediate post-transfusion platelet count to be >30,000/uL and the 24 hour platelet count to be >20,000/uL.

Overt bleeding will be controlled in nearly all thrombocytopenic patients if the posttransfusion platelet count is 40,000/uL or higher. In contrast, bleeding diminishes in only about one third of patients when the posttransfusion platelet count remains <20,000/uL. If the posttransfusion platelet count is not sustained, bleeding will resume when the platelet count falls below 10,000/uL. Therefore, the platelet count needs to be maintained above 10,000 to 20,000/uL for at least 24 hours.

Refractoriness
Alloimmunization against histocompatibility antigens occurs in 25 to 35% of patients with acute leukemia who are transfused with multiple random donor platelet transfusions and in 4 to 5% transfused with apheresis platelets. This is the most important long-term complication of platelet transfusions because patients become refractory to future platelet transfusions.

- An adult patient is considered to be refractory if the 10-60 minute post-transfusion platelet count fails to rise more than 2000/uL per random platelet concentrate or 10,000 to 12,000/uL per apheresis platelet.

- Children are considered to be refractory if the one hour post-tranfusion platelet count fails to rise more than 3500/uL per random donor platelet concentrate.

- Because patients may have a poor post-transfusion increment to a single transfusion yet have excellent platelet increments with subsequent transfusions, a diagnosis of refractoriness should only be made when at least two ABO compatible transfusions, stored less than 72 hours, result in poor increments.

Other causes of platelet destruction should also be ruled out including:

- Fever
- Sepsis,
- Splenomegaly
- DIC
- Bleeding
- Status post-BMT
- Alloimmunization
- Drug induced immune thrombocytopenia.

The diagnosis of refractoriness should be confirmed by testing for platelet antibody, which detects antibody to HLA and platelet-specific antigens. Approximately 90% of alloimmunized patients will have demonstrable platelet antibody.

If the platelet antibody test is positive, a refractory patient is best managed by transfusion of crossmatch compatible apheresis platelets. There is no evidence that alloimmunized patients benefit from continued prophylactic transfusion of incompatible platelets that do not produce an increase in posttransfusion platelet count.

If there is an inadequate post transfusion platelet count increment following 4 consecutive crossmatch compatible single donor platelets, it is reasonable to revert to the use of randomly selected products. It is important to obtain platelet counts 10 minutes to 1 hour following each transfusion of compatible platelets since a useful but temporary post transfusion increment may occur but be missed if platelet counts are not obtained until the next morning.

Bleeding patients, for whom compatible platelet donors cannot be found in a timely manner, may benefit from repeated transfusions of pooled random donor platelets (10 or more concentrates per pool). Large numbers of random platelets may adsorb much of the platelet antibody and fortuitously include some compatible units. Intravenous immune globulin and plasma exchanges are not effective in reducing the refractory state.

If the platelet antibody screening test is negative, refractoriness is probably due to clinical factors rather than alloimmunization and crossmatched platelets will not be beneficial .

PLASMA

Three plasma products are generally available today: Fresh Frozen Plasma (FFP), Plasma frozen within 24 hours after Phlebotomy (FP24) and Thawed Plasma. All of these products are usually prepared from a unit of whole blood, but may also be collected by apheresis. Each bag of plasma prepared from whole blood has a volume between 175 and 250 mL. Plasma prepared by apheresis contains a volume of 400 to 600 mL.

The major difference between FFP and FP24 is that FFP is separated from a unit of whole blood and frozen at -18°C within 8 hours after collection, whereas a unit of FP24 is frozen within 8 to 24 hours after collection. Both products can be stored frozen for up to 1 year and expire 24 hours after thawing. Because of the delay in freezing, the Factor VIII content of FP24 is 20 to 40% lower than the pre-storage concentration, compared to a 10 to 20% decrease for FFP. The decreased level of Factor VIII does not prevent FP24 from correcting a coagulopathy because the Factor VIII concentration of the unit remains above the minimal hemostatic level of 30% and many patients have elevated Factor VIII levels because it is an acute phase reactant.

If a unit of FFP or FP24 is not transfused within 24 hours after thawing, it can be relabeled as Thawed Plasma and stored for an additional 4 days at 1 to 6°C. The FDA has not issued guidance on conversion of FP24 to Thawed Plasma, but this appears to be common practice. All coagulation factors are maintained at relatively normal levels, except for Factor VIII which declines to 40% of the prestorage level. Conversion of FFP or FP24 decreases product wastage and improves turnaround time in emergency situations because it has already been thawed and can be issued immediately.

Pre-transfusion crossmatching of plasma is not necessary. Units of FFP should be ABO compatible whenever possible. Alternative ABO groups may be substituted as long as the recipients' red blood cells are compatible with anti-A or B antibodies present in the donor plasma. The following table provides guidelines for selection of compatible FFP units:

ABO Compatible FFP

Recipient ABO Group	Compatible FFP
O	O, A, B, AB
A	A, AB
B	B, AB
AB	AB

FFP Transfusion Guidelines

General guidelines for FFP transfusion include:

1. Treatment of a coagulopathy prior to an invasive procedure
2. Treatment of a coagulopathy in a patient who is bleeding
3. Plasma exchange for thrombotic thrombocytopenic purpura (TTP)
4. Prophylactic treatment for patients with hereditary angioedema

Today, much plasma is ordered prophylactically to correct an elevated protime (PT) prior to an invasive procedure. Physicians performing invasive procedures want to avoid hemorrhagic complications and often regard a mild elevation of a coagulation test result as an indication to order plasma. The decision to prophylactically transfuse plasma is based on three unproven assumptions:

1. Mild prolongation of PT/INR (defined as an INR <1.7) predicts bleeding from an invasive procedure
2. Pre-procedure transfusion of plasma will correct a prolonged PT/INR
3. Prophylactic plasma transfusions result in fewer bleeding events.
   The evidence clearly contradicts the first assumption. PT and APTT begin to rise above the upper limit of the normal range when coagulation factor levels fall below approximately 70% of normal. When the INR increases to 1.3 - 1.5, vitamin K dependent coagulation factors are still 50% of normal. Even at an INR between 1.8 and 2.0, they remain at 30% of normal, which is still at or above the minimal hemostatic level of 20 -30%. These results explain why a mildly elevated PT/INR is not usually associated with spontaneous hemorrhage and does not increase the risk of bleeding during routine invasive procedures. Studies during the last 20 years in patients undergoing liver biopsies, bronchoscopic biopsies, renal biopsies, central line vein cannulation, thoracentesis and angiography have repeatedly demonstrated that PT and activated plasma thromboplastin time (APTT) are not predictive of hemorrhage. However, it must be remembered that the risk of bleeding is greater if the platelet count is decreased, platelet function is abnormal, or the patient has experienced massive trauma or is undergoing extensive surgery.

Additional evidence clearly disputes assumptions 2 and 3. Prophylactic transfusion of plasma to correct a mildly elevated INR prior to an invasive procedure is often not effective. When the INR is <1.7, transfusion of plasma corrects INR an average of only 0.1 per unit transfused, largely because the INR of plasma itself ranges between 1.0 and 1.3. The difference in coagulation activity between donor plasma and patient plasma is so small that plasma transfusions produce minimal demonstrable effect on the patient's INR.

INR Correction by FFP

Pre-transfusion INR	Correction per FFP unit Mean & Range
1.3 - 1.7	0.1 (0.1 - 0.2)
1.7 - 2.3	0.2 (0.1 - 0.3)
2.4 - 2.9	0.4 (0.1 - 0.7)
3.0 - 4.3	0.7 (0.2 - 1.5)
4.4 - 20.0	3.5 (1.1 - 8.4)

While a patient with an INR of 1.7 or less may bleed during an invasive procedure, the medical literature clearly demonstrates that the incidence of hemorrhage is not different from that of patients with a normal INR.

In summary, plasma transfusion has minimal effect on normalizing the INR in patients with mildly prolonged INRs for the following reasons:

- Plasma produced from healthy blood donors can have an INR as high as 1.3
- Plasma transfusion to a patient with an INR of less than 1.7 has minimal effect
- Plasma transfusion to patients with an INR of less than 1.7 does not decrease the INR more than usual medical care without plasma transfusion

In view of this information, the common practice of prescribing plasma to correct a mildly elevated INR prior to an invasive procedure needs to be reevaluated. It is not necessary or efficacious to correct an INR below 1.7 to achieve adequate hemostasis.

For patients with highly prolonged INR secondary to excessive anticoagulation, the American College of Chest Physicians (ACCP) has published guidelines to facilitate warfarin reversal in patients with or without bleeding.

ACCP Warfarin Reversal Guidelines

INR	Treatment Recommendations
<5	Withhold warfarin until INR therapeutic
>5 & <9	Withhold 1 or 2 doses Give 2.5 mg Vitamin K orally, especially if patient is at risk of bleeding. For rapid reversal for surgery, give 2.5-5.0 mg Vitamin K orally
>9	Hold warfarin & give 5 mg Vitamin K orally
>20	Hold warfarin & give 10 mg Vitamin K SC or IV & FFP

For elective surgery, the best strategy for warfarin reversal is to discontinue warfarin 3 to 5 days prior to the procedure. Patients presenting with minor bleeding may be treated by withholding the next dose of warfarin and giving oral Vitamin K. When vitamin K replacement therapy is used, its effect does not begin until 6-12 hours after administration and is not complete until 36 hours. Patients with greatly elevated INR's are at high risk for intracranial hemorrhage and should be given plasma concomitantly with vitamin K therapy.

Acquired abnormalities of hemostasis may occur with a variety of other clinical disorders. These usually involve multiple plasma coagulation factor deficits and are more common than inherited plasma deficiencies that usually involve single coagulation factor deficiencies. Consequently, there is a concurrent derangement of several coagulation tests as shown in following table.

Acquired Plasma Coagulopathies

Condition	Coagulation Defect
Liver disease – mild	Abnormal PT
Liver disease –moderate to severe	Abnormal PT, PTT, D-Dimer, platelet function
Acute DIC	PT, PTT, low platelet count, low fibrinogen, elevated D-Dimer
Postoperative bleeding	Minimal PT & PTT elevation, low platelet count
Massive Transfusion	Minimal PT & PTT elevation, low platelet count
Vitamin K deficiency, mild	Abnormal PT (decreased factor VII)
Vitamin K deficiency, moderate to severe	Abnormal PT & aPTT (decreased II, VII, IX, X)

The goal of plasma transfusion is to increase the plasma level of each coagulation factor above 30%. Each bag increases the level of any coagulation factor 2 to 3% and fibrinogen 8 mg/dL in an average adult. A dose of 10 to 15 mL of plasma per kg body weight will increase coagulation factors by 8 to 10%, while a dose of 30 to 35 mL per kg body weight will increase them by 30 to 35%. The lower dose corresponds to 3 to 6 bags of plasma in an average 70 kg adult, while the higher dose corresponds to 8 to 14 bags. The PT and PTT should be rechecked before subsequent units are transfused. If the PT and PTT remain prolonged, more plasma may be indicated.

FFP is the treatment of choice for congenital factor deficiencies when more specific concentrates are not available. Examples include factors V and XI.

Congenital Coagulation Factor Deficiencies

Coagulation Factor	Deficiency Prevalence	Minimal Hemostatic Level	Circulating Half-Life	Preferred Component
I fibrinogen	Very Rare	100 mg/dL	3 - 5 days	Cryoprecipitate
II prothrombin	Very Rare	20 - 40%	2 - 5 days	Prothrombin Complex
V	1 per million births	25%	15 - 36 hours	FFP
VII	1 per 500,000 births	10 - 20%	4 - 7 hours	Recombinant VIIa (Novoseven)
VIII	1 per 5,000 male births	30%	9 - 18 hours	Recombinant Factor VIII concentrate
vWF	1 per 1,000 births	25 - 50%	Few hours	Factor VIII concentrate with vWF
IX	1 per 30,000 male births	25 - 50%	20 - 24 hours	Prothrombin concentrate
X	1 per 500,000 births	10 - 25%	32 - 48 hours	Prothrombin complex
XI	4% Ashkenazi Jews	15 - 25%	2.5 - 3.5 days	FFP
XIII	1 per several million births	5%	7 days	Cryoprecipitate

Dosing of plasma for congenital factor deficiencies is dependent upon the degree of factor deficiency and the half-life of the deficient factor(s). All of the factors noted above, except V and VII, have a half-life greater than 12 hours and do not need to be replaced more often than every 12 hours. A practical approach for an average adult would be to give:

- Initial loading dose of 4 units of plasma prior to surgery
- Maintenance dose of 2 units of plasma every 12 hours
- Measure factor level after 24 hours
- Readjust dose as needed

Plasma may be needed for massive transfusions of greater than one blood volume in patients who have a demonstrable coagulopathy and continued bleeding. Thrombocytopenia is responsible for continued bleeding during massive transfusion more often than coagulation factor depletion. Platelet transfusion should be tried first if the platelet count is <50,000/uL. Current massive transfusion guidelines recommend a 1 to 1 ratio of RBCs and plasma.

Plasma is indicated for the treatment of Thrombotic Thrombocytopenic Purpura (TTP) and hemolytic uremic syndrome (HUS). Plasma can be given as a continuous infusion or during plasma exchange. Continuous infusion is not recommended because of its increased risk of fluid overload. A single plasma exchange, which replaces approximately 60% of a patient's plasma volume, usually requires 10 to 12 units of plasma.

Plasma can be used for prophylaxis in patients with hereditary angioedema who are undergoing oral surgery. Prophylaxis will prevent attacks of angioedema which are commonly precipitated by dental procedures and head and neck surgery. Infusion of 2 units of FFP the day before and again just prior to the procedure is recommended. Although FFP is recommended for prophylaxis, its use for treatment of an angioedema attack has not been established. Plasma transfusions have been reported to arrest attacks of angioedema. However, FFP could be hazardous because it contains complement factors C2 and C4 that may exacerbate the attack. FFP should be reserved for life threatening attacks. Future treatment options include C1 Inhibitor concentrates that have been used for years in Europe and are currently under clinical investigation in the United States.

FFP should not be used as a volume expander, as a nutritional supplement, for the treatment of bleeding in the absence of documented coagulopathy, or as a standing order following surgery or massive transfusion.

It is important to remember that transfusion of FFP is not free of risk. FFP is the blood component most frequently associated with transfusion-related acute lung injury (TRALI). Today, TRALI is one of the most common causes of a fatal transfusion reaction. As with any other blood component, the decision to transfuse FFP should be based on predictable benefit and clinically necessity.

CRYOPRECIPITATE

Cryoprecipitate refers to the proteins that precipitate out of solution when a unit of fresh frozen plasma is slowly thawed in the cold at 1 to 6°C and then refrozen within one hour. Each bag contains Factor VIII, fibrinogen, von Willebrand factor, and Factor XIII suspended in 10 to 15 mL of residual plasma. Bags are stored at –18°C or colder. Since several bags of cryoprecipitate are transfused at a time, the transfusion service or blood center pools them into a sterile plastic transfer pack and stores them at 20-24°C until administration. Cryoprecipitate outdates 6 hours after being thawed or 4 hours after being pooled. ABO compatible cryoprecipitate is desirable if large volumes will be transfused, but Rh compatibility is not important because no red blood cells are present. Cryoprecipitate should be infused through a standard blood filter at a rate of 4 to 10 mL/minute. At this rate, a pool of 10 bags can be infused in approximately 30 minutes. The risk of viral transmission from cryoprecipitate is the same as other plasma products.

Indications & Dose

Conversion of fibrinogen into fibrin is the last stage of the coagulation sequence. Fibrinogen plays an important role in fibrin clot formation and platelet aggregation. If fibrinogen is decreased, bleeding may ensue.

Acquired hypofibrinogenemia is most commonly associated with:

- Severe liver disease
- Head trauma
- Acute DIC
- Tissue plasminogen activator (TPA) therapy
- Streptokinase & urokinase therapy
- Chemotherapy with asparaginase
- Plasma exchange with albumin

The transfusion service often receives orders for fresh frozen plasma (FFP) to treat the prolonged protime (PT) and activated partial thromboplastin time (aPTT) associated with hypofibrinogenemia. Although FFP contains fibrinogen, it is not the optimal blood component because of the very large volumes of plasma that are required to increase fibrinogen to hemostatic levels. Cryoprecipitate is preferred because it contains the same concentration of fibrinogen as FFP in less than one-twentieth of the volume.

Cryoprecipitate should be given when the fibrinogen level falls below 100 mg/dL, which is the minimal level needed for hemostasis. Each bag of cryoprecipitate contains 200 to 250 mg of fibrinogen and will increase the plasma fibrinogen level of a 70-kg adult by 6 to 8 mg/dL. Generally, 10 bags of cryoprecipitate are given if the fibrinogen level is between 50 and 100 mg/dL and 20 bags are given if it is less than 50 mg/dL. A fibrinogen level should be measured at 30 to 60 minutes after completion of the transfusion to determine if additional doses are needed. The therapeutic goal is to keep the plasma fibrinogen level above 100 mg/dL. The circulating half life of fibrinogen is 3 to 5 days.

Cryoprecipitate may be given prophylactically for head trauma because of the associated disseminated intravascular coagulation that can result in intracranial hemorrhage. In patients with either blunt or penetrating head trauma, 10 units of cryoprecipitate may be given empirically or when serial fibrinogen levels indicate a precipitous drop in fibrinogen level.

Cryoprecipitate should be transfused to patients with congenital fibrinogen deficiency only when they are bleeding or prior to an invasive or surgical procedure. Cryoprecipitate is the treatment of choice for patients with documented factor XIII deficiency whom are actively bleeding or undergoing an invasive or surgical procedure. Factor XIII deficiency can usually be treated with 1 bag of cryoprecipitate for every 10 kg of body weight. Factor XIII assays should be used to evaluate the need for repeat administration in Factor XIII deficiency.

Cryoprecipitate is beneficial in correcting the thrombopathy associated with uremia. Ten bags of cryoprecipitate are usually required to reverse a qualitative platelet defect. The maximum therapeutic effect takes at least 4 hours after infusion to develop and lasts approximately 24 hours. Repeat administration of cryoprecipitate provides limited improvement. The use of cryoprecipitate to correct a qualitative platelet defect should be reserved for life-threatening hemorrhage or prior to an invasive procedure. Alternatively, dialysis can be used to correct the uremic platelet defect.

Cryoprecipitate can also be used as a local hemostatic sealant and this application is commonly referred to as fibrin glue. It is best used when cautery and suture cannot control localized bleeding. Diffuse bleeding will not improve with fibrin glue. The three essential ingredients of fibrin sealant are the fibrinogen present in cryoprecipitate, bovine or human thrombin, and calcium chloride. A vial of lyophilized thrombin is reconstituted with calcium chloride and aspirated into one chamber of a double-barreled syringe. One or two units of cryoprecipitate are generally used as a fibrin sealant depending on the severity of the bleeding and the surface area to be covered. A single unit of cryoprecipitate is aspirated into the other barrel. Both solutions are delivered simultaneously through a blunt tipped cannula or spray atomizer on to the bleeding site. A clot forms in a matter of seconds to minutes, and lasts up to 2 weeks. Adverse effects include the formation of antibodies to bovine thrombin and factor V, which may cause bleeding. Another potential complication is anaphylaxis.

Cryoprecipitate should not be used to treat von Willebrand's disease except in life and limb-threatening emergencies when multimeric vWF-containing Factor VIII concentrate (Humate P, Alphanate, or Koate DVI) is not immediately available. A reasonable dose of cryoprecipitate is 1 bag for every 10 Kg of body weight. This dose should be repeated every 8 to 12 hours. The amount of von Willebrand factor contained within a given unit of cryoprecipitate is highly variable and dependent upon the donor's plasma level.

Cryoprecipitate should be used to treat Hemophilia A only when Factor VIII concentrate is not available. Cryoprecipitate should never be used for the treatment of hemophilia B since it lacks Factor IX.

SPECIAL BLOOD PRODUCTS

Leukocyte-Reduced Red Cells and Platelets
Units of whole blood, red blood cells, and platelets contain significant numbers of leukocytes while fresh frozen plasma and cryoprecipitate do not. Transfusion of leukocytes has been associated with several adverse sequelae, including:

- Febrile transfusion reactions
- Transfusion related acute lung injury (TRALI)
- HLA alloimmunization of chronically transfused patients
- Refractoriness to platelet transfusions
- Leukotropic (CMV and HTLV) virus transmission
- Immune suppression
- Graft vs. Host Disease

Leukocytes can be removed immediately after collection or at the bedside using third generation adsorption filters that remove 99.9% of leukocytes. Pre-storage leukoreduction has the additional advantages of preventing cytokine release from white blood cells during storage and elimination of the need for bedside filters that have slower flow rates than standard blood filters. Prestorage leukocyte reduction has also been proven to more consistently remove enough white blood cells to meet the definition of a leukocyte reduced unit. If bedside leukoreduction is necessary, one unit of red blood cells can be transfused through a single filter. A pool of 8-10 random donor platelet concentrates can be transfused through a single platelet filter.

On September 18, 1998, the Blood Products Advisory Committee of the FDA recommended universal leukoreduction of all cellular blood components, except granulocytes. Many other countries already required universal leukoreduction of blood components.

If a hospital has not implemented universal leukoreduction, leukocyte reduced blood components should be used in the following situations:

Established Indications:

- Prevention of febrile reactions following two documented febrile reactions
- Febrile reaction and demonstrable WBC antibodies
- Prevention of transfusion related acute lung injury
- Prevention of HLA alloimmunization in multi-transfused patients including:
    - Chronic hemolytic anemia
    - Aplastic anemia
    - Myelodysplastic syndromes
    - Myeloproliferative syndromes
- Bone marrow transplant candidates
- Heart transplant recipients
- Substitute for CMV negative components, when none are available
- HIV infected patients
- Antepartum transfusions for CMV negative women

Leukocyte reduced components may also delay or prevent alloimmunization to HLA and leukocyte-specific antigens in chronically transfused patients and, thereby, delay the onset of refractoriness to random donor platelet transfusions. Patients expected to receive only a few blood components, such as during elective surgery, do not derive much benefit from the additional expense.

Some viruses such as CMV reside in granulocytes. Pre-storage leukocyte reduction eliminates the risk of CMV transmission. Leukocyte removal filtration can be used when CMV negative components are not available: Leukocyte reduced units will not prevent graft versus host disease. Plasma components such as FFP and cryoprecipitate do not need to be leukoreduced because they contain so few leukocytes.

Administration of pre-storage leukoreduced RBCs and platelets is the same as regular units. The use of bedside leukoreduction filters may significantly slow flow rates, which precludes their use in emergent situations where multiple rapid transfusions are required. External pressure devices should not be used, because they reduce the efficiency of leukocyte removal.

Saline-Washed Red Blood Cells

Saline-washed RBCs are units of whole blood or RBCs that have been washed with 1 to 2 liters of saline manually or in an automated cell washer. Washed units contain 10 to 20% less RBCs than the original units. Therefore, a greater number of washed units may be required to alleviate symptoms. These units have a hematocrit of 70% and have been depleted of 99% of the plasma proteins and 85% of the leukocytes. The residual potassium concentration is 0.2 mEq/L. Other RBC metabolites are almost entirely removed. Washing also removes cytokines that cause febrile reactions. Saline washed RBCs must be used within 24 h after washing since the original collection bag has been entered, which breaks the hermetic seal and increases the possibility of bacterial contamination. Removal of the anticoagulant-preservative solution also limits cell viability and function. Saline washed red blood cells have limited medical indications.

Indications for Saline Washed Blood Components

1. Febrile transfusion reactions not prevented by leukocyte reduction.
2. IgA deficiency with documented anti-IgA antibodies and IgA deficient donor not available
3. History of a previous anaphylactic transfusion reaction.
4. Severe urticarial reactions not prevented by pre-transfusion antihistamines.

5. Potassium depletion of units irradiated more than 12 hours before that will be transfused to a neonate or fetus.

Administration of IgA containing products to patients with anti-IgA results in anaphylaxis. Washing red cell and platelet components is one modality to prevent anaphylaxis, while transfusion of blood components from IgA deficient donors is another. Most regional blood centers maintain a registry of IgA deficient donors.

Irradiated components have elevated levels of plasma potassium. Washing units with saline can decrease potassium levels. However, the best policy is to irradiate units immediately before transfusion.

Inappropriate use of saline washed whole blood or red blood cells includes:

- Emergent situations because they are not readily available
- Questionable transfusions because units outdate 24 hours after washing
- Non IgA deficient patients
- Febrile reactions that can be successfully treated with antipyretics and leukocyte depleted components.

Administration of washed components is the same as those covered in their respective sections, except for the shortened shelf life of 24 hours. Platelets can also be washed. The major indication is transfusion of maternal apheresis platelets to an infant with neonatal alloimmune thrombocytopenia.

Irradiated Blood Components

Irradiated components are units of RBCs, platelets, and granulocytes that have been gamma irradiated with a dose of 25 Gy to the central portion and a minimum dose of 15 Gy to any portion of the unit. Each component must be labeled with a radiation sensitive label to indicate that an adequate dose of irradiation has been given. Gamma irradiation inactivates lymphocytes and prevents transfusion associated graft versus host disease (GVHD). All cellular blood components should be irradiated including whole blood, red blood cells, platelets, and granulocytes. Leukocyte reduction by filtration does not remove sufficient numbers of lymphocytes to prevent graft versus host disease. Fresh frozen plasma and cryoprecipitate do not need to be irradiated.

Irradiation does not affect cell survival or function but does damage the red blood cell membrane sodium-potassium pump, causing leakage of potassium across the cell membrane into the plasma. Plasma potassium levels increase almost twofold within 24 hours. This potassium load is not harmful to most adults, but could significantly elevate potassium levels in neonates and fetuses due to their small blood volume. This potential problem can be avoided by irradiating units just prior to transfusion. If unforeseen delays occur, the unit can be saline washed to remove potassium.

IRRADIATED BLOOD COMPONENT INDICATIONS

Established Indications:

1. Recipients of bone marrow & hematopoietic stem cell transplants
2. Children with severe congenital T cell deficiencies
3. Fetal transfusions
4. Neonates who received irradiated components as fetuses

5. All granulocyte transfusions

6. Recipients of directed donor transfusions from blood relatives.

7. Exchange transfusions for hemolytic disease of the newborn

8. HLA matched or crossmatched platelet transfusions

9. Recipients with Hodgkin's Disease

Less well established indications:

1. Non-Hodgkin's hematologic malignancies.

2. Premature infants weighing < 1200g.

3. Patients with solid tumors receiving chemotherapy and/or radiation therapy.

Administration of irradiated products is the same as the administration of non-irradiated products.

CMV Negative Blood Components

Transfusion acquired CMV is of little concern in immunocompetent individuals, but can be a serious problem in immunocompromised patients. In the latter group of patients, CMV transmission can result in pneumonitis, chronic hepatitis, gastroenteritis, chorioretinitis, or disseminated disease. CMV negative blood components are indicated for patients in the first two groups in the table below. Indications for CMV negative units have not yet been well established for the third group of patients.

INDICATIONS FOR THE TRANSFUSION CMV NEGATIVE PRODUCTS

Established Indications

1. All fetal and intrauterine transfusions.

2. Low birth weight premature infants born to CMV seronegative mothers.

3. CMV negative recipients of organ, peripheral blood stem cell or bone marrow transplants from CMV negative donors.

4. Antepartum transfusions for CMV negative women.

Less Well Established Indications

1. CMV negative patients with HIV

2. CMV negative patients who are potential candidates for autologous or allogeneic bone marrow transplant.

3. CMV negative patients undergoing splenectomy

4. Potential seronegative donors for bone marrow transplant.

Unestablished Indications

1. CMV negative BMT recipients from CMV positive donors

2. CMV positive BMT recipients

3. CMV negative solid organ transplants from CMV positive donors

4. CMV positive recipients of solid organ transplants

Depending on need, a blood center screens a certain percentage of donated units for CMV IgG and IgM antibody. Seronegative donors serve as a continuous supply of CMV negative products. The CMV status of these donors is reconfirmed with each donation. Administration of CMV negative units is the same as regular units of red blood cells and platelets.

Rh Immune Globulin for Prevention of Hemolytic Disease of the Newborn

RhD hemolytic disease is caused by maternal immunization to the D antigen, followed by subsequent transfer of maternal IgG across the placenta resulting in immune hemolysis of fetal red blood cells. Anti-D is usually not detectable for 5 to 15 weeks after sensitization, which is much slower than the usual immune response to other foreign antigens such as microorganisms. The incidence of maternal alloimmunization in the United States and European Union remains at 1 to 1.5 percent of at risk D negative women despite the introduction of prophylactic RhD immune globulin.

RhD immune globulin (RhIg) is a concentrated solution of IgG anti-D derived from human plasma. A 1 mL full dose vial is sufficient to counteract the immunizing effects of 15 mL of Rh positive red cells. It was developed to prevent immunization of Rh-negative women to the D antigen and thereby prevent hemolytic disease of the newborn (HDN) caused by anti-D.

The following is a summary of RhIg administration guidelines:
- RhIg should be given at 26 to 28 weeks gestation if a woman is D-negative and the antibody screen is negative for anti-D. If the first prenatal visit is earlier than 26 weeks gestation, the antibody screen should be repeated at 26 weeks prior to administration of RhIg.
- RhIg should be given if a woman is D-negative, the antibody screen is positive, and the antibody is not anti-D.
- RhIg should not be given if a woman is D-negative, the antibody screen is positive and the antibody is anti-D.
- RhIg should not be given if a woman is D-positive, regardless of the antibody screen result.
- RhIg is not necessary for women who are weak D positive.

RhIg Administration Guidelines

Rh Type	Antibody Screen	RhIg Administration
D negative	Negative	Yes
D negative	Positive with anti-D	No
D negative	Positive with other antibody	Yes
D positive	Negative	No
D positive	Positive with other antibody	No

D-negative women who have received RhIg antenatally often have subsequent positive antibody screens due to passively acquired anti-D. A selected cell panel should be run to exclude clinically significant alloantibodies other than anti-D. If no other clinically significant alloantibodies are found, except passive anti-D, these pregnancies do not need to be handled as high risk.

RhIg should be administered to all D-negative women with no evidence of anti-D within 72 hours of any event that may increase the risk of FMH such as:
- Pregnancy termination at 13 weeks gestation or later
- Amniocentesis
- Chorionic villus sampling
- PUBS
- External version
- Suspected placental pathology

If the pregnancy is at or after 26 weeks gestation, the need for additional doses of RhIg should be determined by testing maternal blood for the presence of excessive fetal maternal hemorrhage (FMH).

If the delivering facility has a verified record of a negative antibody screen during the current pregnancy, repeat maternal testing is not required at the time of delivery unless a question of HDN arises.

- If the delivering facility has a verified record of immunization to D, RhIg should not be given.
- If the mother is known to be D-negative and not immunized to D and the cord blood types as D negative, RhIg should not be given and no further testing is necessary.
- If the mother is known to be D-negative and not immunized to D and the cord blood types as D positive (including weak D), a test for excessive FMH should be performed to determine RhIg dosage. An appropriate dose of RhIg should be given.
- If the mother is known to be D-negative and not immunized to D and the cord blood is not tested, a test for excessive FMH should be performed to determine RhIg dosage. Either the Kleihauer Betke or flow cytometry method can be utilized. An appropriate dose of RhIg should be administered.

The amount of fetal maternal hemorrhage is calculated by multiplying the percent fetal cells by 50 (maternal blood volume is typically 5 liters or 50 deciliters). This product is then divided by 30, which is the volume of fetal blood neutralized by a single vial of RhIg (300 ug dose).

$$\text{Vials of RhIg} = \% \text{ fetal cells} \times 50/30$$

For example, if the percent of fetal hemorrhage is 2%, then the volume of fetal hemorrhage is 100 mL. Dividing 100 mL by 30 mL/vial yields 3.3 vials. This number is rounded down to 3 and 1 vial is added for insurance. The required dose is 4 vials.

RhIg is very safe and has a very low risk of viral transmission, especially of enveloped viruses. A potential risk of anaphylaxis exists in IgA deficient patients. No more than 5 vials should be injected into each buttock at one time. Large doses should be given at 12-hour intervals over a 72-hour period.

Intravenous RhIg (WinRho™, Rhyphylac®) is also available. Dosage recommendations are the same as for IM RhIg. IV RhIg is preferrable to IM RhIg when large doses are required. Advantages include its rapid effect, less patient discomfort, and larger allowable single dose. The major disadvantage is increased cost.

RhIG therapy should also be considered for Rh-negative women of child bearing age (or female children) who inadvertently or necessarily are exposed to Rh-positive red cells through platelet or red cell transfusions. Dose is based on the estimated packed red cell volume of the component transfused. RhIG therapy should be started as soon as possible after the transfusion event, but may be administered over several days if a large number of vials are needed.

RhIG for Treatment of ITP
Intravenous RhIg (WinRho SDF or Rhophylac) is effective in some patients with immune thrombocytopenia (ITP) including:

- Children with acute or chronic ITP
- Adults with chronic ITP
- Children and adults with HIV-related ITP

Administration of IV RhIG to a Rh positive patient results in the binding of anti-D antibody to the patients' red blood cells. In a thrombocytopenic patient, there are approximately 500 antibody-coated red cells for every antibody-coated platelet. The reticuloendothelial system phagocytizes red cells instead of platelets, allowing the platelet count to increase. This reticuloendothelial Fc receptor blockade has been referred to as a medical splenectomy.

Patients must be Rh positive and have not undergone splenectomy. An initial dose of 250 IU (50 ug) per kg of body weight is recommended unless the hemoglobin level is <10 g/dL. In this situation, a smaller dose of 125 to 200 IU (25 to 40 ug) per kg is indicated. The initial dose can be administered at one time or divided into 2 doses given on separate days. Additional doses of 125 to 300 IU/kg can be given as needed.

A decrease in hemoglobin levels up to 1.7 g/dL is expected because passively administered anti-D attaches to the D antigen on the patient's RBCs and shortens their life span. Some patients experience more severe intravascular hemolysis, which may be life threatening. If a patient needs to be transfused, Rh negative red blood cells should be given to prevent further exacerbation of hemolysis.

Patients treated with IV RhIG will develop a positive direct antiglobulin test and a positive antibody screen. In addition to anti-D, passively acquired anti-D, C and E antibodies may be detected.

If IV RhIg is not available, ITP can be treated with intramuscular RhIg (RhoGam). Doses of 13 ug/kg can be given weekly. One to two days after treatment, the platelet count should rise to approximately 50,000/uL and gradually peak at 7-14 days.

Fibrin Sealant
On May 1,1998, FDA approved the first commercially available fibrin sealant for use as an adjunct to hemostasis in surgery. The same product is available from two different distributors with the trade names of Tisseel and Hemasell APR. More recently, the FDA approved a second generation fibrin sealant with the trade name of Evicel (Ethicon) for use in general surgery. A single vial contains fibrinogen, thrombin, aprotinin, and calcium carbonate. The advantages of Tisseel over cryoprecipitate include lower risk of viral transmission and more consistent batch to batch potency. The major clinical applications include colostomy closures, CABG, and splenic trauma. Pharmacy rather than the Blood Bank usually stocks this product.

Recombinant FVIIa
Recombinant Factor VIIa (rFVIIa, NovoSeven) received FDA approval for the treatment of bleeding in hemophilia patients with inhibitors to Factor VIII or Factor IX on April 19, 1999. More recently, it has been used off-label for a variety of bleeding disorders. Factor VIIa complexes with tissue factor at the site of injury and induces activation of Factor X, resulting in clot formation.

Supraphysiologic doses of rFVIIa bind directly to tissue factor that is exposed on damaged endothelium and directly activates Factor X, bypassing the intrinsic pathway of coagulation. It also binds directly to thrombin activated platelets.

Recombinant Factor VIIa is supplied in three sizes: 1.2, 2.4 and 4.8 mg per vial. The product is supplied as a freeze-dried powder that is reconstituted in sterile water. It should be administered by IV push over a period of one to two minutes within 3 hours after reconstitution.

Currently, there is no satisfactory laboratory test to monitor the clinical effectiveness of rFVIIa. Protime and aPTT shorten, but do not necessarily reflect clinical effectiveness.

Recombinant FVIIa is appropriate for management of acute hemorrhage in hemophilia patients with high-titer inhibitors (>5 BU). The recommended dose of rFVIIa is 90 ug/kg by IV bolus given every two hours for 24 hours or until hemostasis is achieved. Once the patient is stabilized, the interval between treatments can be lengthened to 3–6 hours. This dosage schedule can be used for patients undergoing major surgery or treatment of serious CNS, intraperitoneal, retroperitoneal or intramuscular (compartment syndrome) bleeding.

For major surgery, a dose of 90 to 120 ug/kg is given every 2 hours for the first 48 hours. The dose can often be decreased to every 4 hours during the third and fourth postoperative days and then to every 6 hours for another week.

A dosage of 90 ug/kg corresponds to plasma levels of 2 ug per mL, assuming 100% recovery. The goal of therapy is to increase peak levels of FVII functional clotting activity (FVII: C), measured immediately after the initial dose, to above 30 U/mL and preferably between 60 and 90 U/mL. Steady state levels measured 2 hours after 90 ug/kg NovoSeven administration following two days of dosing at 2-hour intervals average 28 U/mL. The protime shortens significantly and often plateaus around 7 seconds. The aPTT may shorten as much as 15 to 20 seconds, but usually does not completely normalize.

An advantage of Factor VIIa is its lower risk of DIC. However, DIC may occur if a patient is first treated with activated prothrombin complex concentrate (APCC) and then switched to rFVIIa. DIC can be prevented by waiting several hours between discontinuing APCC and starting rFVIIa infusions.

FVII deficiency is a rare coagulation disorder that may be associated with spontaneous bleeding episodes in severely deficient patients or bleeding after surgery in mildly affected patients.

- If the patient's plasma FVII level is >25%, they can usually be managed with 15 mL/kg of FFP. Factor VIIa may be necessary if the patient is undergoing cardiothoracic, neurologic, ophthalmologic, or trauma surgery.

- If the patients plasma FVII level is <25% and they are undergoing minor surgery, they should be initially treated with 15 mL/kg of FFP. Doses of 5 mL/kg of FFP can be repeated at 6 hour intervals until hemostasis is achieved.

- If the patient's plasma FVII level is <25% and they have a serious bleeding episode or are undergoing cardiothoracic, neurologic, ophthalmologic, or trauma surgery, they should be treated initially with rFVIIa at a dose of 15 – 30 ug/kg every 2 hours until hemostasis is achieved. Once bleeding is controlled, this dose can be administered every 6 to 12 hours as needed. This dose corresponds to a 1.2 mg vial for a 70 kg adult.

rFVIIa has been used to treat patients with factor XI deficiency either with or without an inhibitor. Doses of 90 to 120 ug/kg every 2 to 3 hours until bleeding has ceased have been effective.

Patients with Glanzman's thrombasthenia have been successfully treated with rFVIIa for surgical prophylaxis or to control excessive menstrual bleeding. This therapy is especially effective for those patients who have developed platelet alloantibody from previous platelet transfusions. The dosage needed to control hemostasis has varied from 90 to120 ug/kg.

Patients undergoing extensive surgery and patients bleeding after severe trauma develop multiple hemostatic defects. Coagulation factors and platelets are both consumed and diluted by massive transfusion and infusion of volume expanders. Coagulation is impaired by hypothermia and acidosis Patients should first be transfused with platelets, FFP, cryoprecipitate and RBCs.

Factor VII is the first vitamin K dependent coagulation factor to be decreased by warfarin. Sometimes patients require urgent reversal of their prolonged INR for an intracerebral hemorrhage. Patients with life threatening or intracranial bleeding can be treated with 20 mL/kg of FFP and a single dose of rFVIIa. A single dose of 80 ug/kg given within 4 hours after the onset of symptoms reduces hematoma growth but does not improve mortality

Off label use of rFVIIa has been associated with thromboembolic events, especially within the first 24 hours after the last dose. Many of the patients who experienced an adverse event were elderly with existing atherosclerotic disease. Thromboembolic events included cerebrovascular, acute myocardial infarction, other arterial thrombosis, pulmonary embolism, other venous thrombosis, and clotted devices.

CHAPTER 9:
Transfusion Therapy for Specific Clinical Situations
WARM AUTOIMMUNE HEMOLYTIC ANEMIA

Autoimmune hemolytic anemias (AIHA) are caused by autoantibodies directed against a patient's own red blood cells that result in accelerated red cell destruction. This disorder is relatively uncommon, with an incidence of 1 in 80,000 individuals. All ages are affected, with the peak incidence occurring in the fourth and fifth decades. Women are more often affected then men.

AIHA are divided into warm and cold autoantibody types based on the temperatures at which the antibodies maximally react with red blood cells in vitro. Warm autoantibodies are more reactive at 37°C than at lower temperatures, whereas cold autoantibodies react optimally at 5°C and less strongly at higher temperatures. These two principal types are further subdivided into primary, or idiopathic, and secondary forms which are associated with an underlying disease. Lymphoproliferative disorders are present in about half of the secondary warm and cold AIHA. Systemic lupus erythematosis and other autoimmune diseases account for the majority of the remaining warm types. Transient cold AIHA are associated with infections, especially mycoplasma pneumonia and infectious mononucleosis.

The clinical picture of warm type AIHA is highly variable. Most patients seek treatment for symptoms attributable to anemia, but occasionally massive hemolysis is seen at onset. Physical findings are related to the degree of anemia and include pallor, resting tachycardia, mild jaundice and occasionally fever. The spleen is usually only mildly enlarged.

Several common laboratory results suggest hemolysis. Hemoglobin is decreased, but the degree of anemia depends on the compensatory capacity of the bone marrow. Reticulocyte count is usually elevated and may result in a mildly elevated MCV. Spherocytes in the peripheral blood smear indicate ongoing red cell destruction. Unconjugated bilirubin is usually, but not always, elevated and urine urobilinogen is increased. Lactate dehydrogenase is usually elevated into the thousands. Serum haptoglobin levels are reduced or undetectable. Hemoglobinemia and hemoglobinuria are present in cases of severe hemolysis. Mild leukocytosis and thrombocytosis may be present.

The diagnosis of AIHA depends on the demonstration of a positive direct antiglobulin test (DAT), indicating the presence of immunoglobulin and/or complement on red blood cells. In warm autoimmune hemolytic anemia, red cells may be coated with IgG, IgG and complement, or complement alone. In warm AIHA, IgG is found alone in about 60% of cases and in association with complement in about 30% of cases. In contrast, cold autoimmune hemolytic anemia is caused by complement-fixing IgM antibodies that react more strongly in the cold than at higher temperatures. In these cases, the direct antiglobulin test detects only complement. Autoantibodies may appear to have specificity for a particular blood group antigen even though the patients' red cells express that antigen.

The strength of the DAT does not predict the severity of disease. For instance, some patients with a strongly positive DAT have little hemolysis, while other patients with a weakly positive DAT hemolyze extensively. Also, the strength of the DAT often does not change following treatment, even though the clinical condition greatly improves.

Transfusion of patients with autoimmune hemolytic anemia is associated with unique risks. Autoantibody often complicates compatibility testing and makes it difficult to exclude the presence of co-existing alloantibodies, thus increasing the risk of a hemolytic transfusion reaction. Approximately 30% of patients with AIHA have detectable alloantibodies. Undetected alloantibodies may cause increased hemolysis following transfusion, which may be mistakenly attributed to an increase in the severity of AIHA. In patients with severe hemolytic anemia, time may be too short to rule out alloantibodies prior to transfusion. In these situations, it is important to remember that alloantibodies typically cause delayed serologic or hemolytic reactions and should be regarded as a tolerable risk in any patient likely to die from rapidly worsening hemolytic anemia.

The autoantibody itself may shorten the survival of transfused red cells. If possible, red blood cell transfusion should be avoided. However, a patient with life threatening anemia should never be denied blood even though the crossmatch is incompatible. If the hemoglobin level is above 8 g/dL, transfusion is rarely necessary or desireable. Clinical judgement is most important at a hemoglobin level between 5 and 8 g/dL. At this level of hemoglobin, many patients with AIHA should be transfused unless close observation indicates that the anemia is not becoming progressively more severe and the patient does not have critical symptoms of anemia. Special consideration should be given to adults greater than 50 years of age with cardiovascular disease. When the hemoglobin falls below 5 g/dL, most patients will require transfusion. The onset of confusion in a patient with worsening anemia is an important clinical indication that transfusion is immediately required.

Warm autoantibodies may demonstrate relative specificity, especially for Rh antigens. Some laboratories select those ABO compatible RBC units that react least strongly with the patient's autoantibody for transfusion. This practice of selecting "least incompatible" units of RBCs has never been proven to provide clinical benefit and should be abandoned because it only delays transfusion. Unusual cases of warm AIHA may react more strongly with a specific antigen, such as Rh e. Insufficient data is available to determine whether providing antigen negative blood in these cases will lessen the risk of alloimmunization or improve red cell survival.

A critical aspect of transfusing patients with AIHA is to avoid over- transfusion. The kinetics of red cell destruction always describe an exponential decay curve, indicating that the number of cells removed during a unit of time is a percentage of the number of cells present at the start of this time interval. Raising the hemoglobin level abruptly is likely to increase the amount of hemolysis that is occurring and may precipitate DIC. Indeed, the most common cause of post transfusion hemoglobinemia and hemoglobinuria in AIHA may not be alloantibody induced hemolysis but rather the quantitative effect of increasing the red cell mass subjected to ongoing autoantibody hemolysis. Accordingly, transfusion of comparatively small volumes of blood is the optimal means of minimizing the danger of transfusion-induced intravascular hemolysis. The patient's hemoglobin level should be maintained just above a tolerable level until more specific therapy becomes effective.

MASSIVE TRANSFUSION

Massive blood loss is defined as the loss of one blood volume within a 24 hour period, a 50% blood volume loss within 3 hours or a rate of loss of 150 mL/minute. The most important factor in the management of hypovolemic shock is to restore the circulating blood volume as rapidly as possible. Blood volume may initially be restored with crystalloid and colloid solutions. Hypothermia increases the risk of end organ failure and coagulopathy and may be prevented by prewarming resuscitation fluids, patient warming devices such as warm air blankets and the use of temperature controlled blood warmers.

When blood loss and fluid replacement reach 40% of blood volume, transfusion of red cells is required. As soon as the need for massive transfusion is recognized, blood samples should be obtained for emergency laboratory tests including ABO and Rh type, antibody screen, compatibility testing, hemoglobin, platelet count, prothrombin time, partial thromboplastin time and fibrinogen. Accurate patient identification is of paramount importance during an emergency situation.

In cases of trauma in which the blood group of the patient is not known it may be necessary to start the transfusion with group O blood while the ABO group is ascertained. Up to 4 units of 0 negative RBC's can be issued before a patient's blood type can be determined. Females of childbearing age should receive O negative RBCs whenever possible to avoid sensitization and the risk of hemolytic disease of the newborn in a subsequent pregnancy. In order to conserve limited supplies of O negative blood, some transfusion services my elect to supply O positive RBCs to older females and males until their blood type is determined. Type specific RBC's may be issued until crossmatches are completed. It takes approximately 30 minutes to have crossmatch compatible blood available after a specimen is received, if the patient has no irregular antibodies.

If a patient with multiple alloantibodies is being massively transfused, >10 units of RBCs have been transfused and the supply of antigen negative RBCs has been exhausted, it may become necessary to switch to partially matched or unmatched blood with the approval of the medical director of the transfusion service. The operating room should immediately be informed of this decision. Antigen typing should be prioritized as described below.

1. Ignore clinically insignificant antibodies such as P^1, Lewis, M, N or Lu^a

2. Ignore historical antibodies that are not currently detectable, except for complement fixing antibodies such as Kidd

3. Ignore clinically significant antibodies that are unlikely to fix complement such as Rh, S, s and Duffy

4. If possible, try to find antigen negative units for antibodies that fix complement such as Kidd

The transfusion service should try to set aside 10 units of antigen negative RBCs for transfusion after the patient's condition has stabilized. Once operating room personnel have informed the transfusion service that bleeding has been controlled, antigen negative units should be issued.

Hemoglobin level should be monitored frequently, with the realization that hemoglobin level is a poor indicator of blood loss in acute bleeding situations. RBC transfusion is rarely needed when the hemoglobin is >9 g/dL, but almost always indicated when it is <7 g/dL. Transfusion should be based on the patient's hemodynamic status.

Plasma may be needed for massive transfusions of greater than one blood volume in patients who have a demonstrable coagulopathy and continued bleeding. The goal is to maintain the INR <1.5 and the aPTT less than 1.5 times the upper limit of the normal range. Thrombocytopenia is responsible for continued bleeding during massive transfusion more often than coagulation factor depletion. Platelet transfusions should be given to maintain the platelet count above 50,000/uL. A higher platelet count may be required with central nervous system injury. Current massive transfusion guidelines recommend a 1:1:1 ratio of RBCs, plasma and platelets. A common practice is to issue 6 units of RBCs, 6 units of plasma and 1 single donor platelet or 6 random donor platelets in a trauma pack. Some transfusion services at trauma centers keep 4 units of group O plasma and 4 units of group A plasma in the thawed state at all times to decrease turnaround time. If it is necessary to supply plasma and platelets before a patient's blood type is known, group AB components are preferred.

Ten units of cryoprecipitate should be given in addition to FFP if the fibrinogen level is <100 mg/dL and 20 units should be given if the fibrinogen is <50 mg/dL. Fibrinogen level should be maintained above 100 mgdL. The need for additional blood components should be assessed by clinical response and repeated laboratory tests.

Occasionally, recombinant factor VIIa (Novoseven) is ordered when the surgeon determines that life threatening coagulaopathic bleeding is present that cannot be surgically corrected. A dose of 90 to 100 ug/kg of rFVIIa may be helpful. If bleeding has not decreased significantly within 30 to 60 minutes, a second dose of 100 ug/kg may be tried. Correction of the pH to greater than 7.2 and correction of hypothermia are recommended prior to rFVIIa infusion because of the markedly decreased activity of rFVIIa in acidosis and hypothermia.

SICKLE CELL DISEASE

Sickle cells are prematurely removed from the circulation by the spleen, resulting in hemolytic anemia. The circulating half life of sickle cells is 16 to 20 days, which is much less than the normal half life of 120 days for normal RBCs.

RBC transfusion provides many benefits including increasing the patient's hemoglobin, diluting the concentration of Hgb S with Hgb A and providing RBCs longer circulating half times that do not sickle nor polymerize. In addition, transfusion suppresses the patient's own erythropoiesis, reducing production of sickle RBCs.

RBCs can be transfused as a simple transfusion or via exchange transfusion. A simple transfusion involves transfusing one or two units of RBCs through a peripheral IV. Exchange transfusion is usually performed using an automated apheresis machine that replaces one to two patient RBC volumes with donor RBCs.

Indications for transfusion in sickle cell disease include:
- Aplastic Crisis
- Stroke
- Splenic Sequestration
- Pregnancy with complications of sickle cell disease
- Priapism if not responsive to hydration and analgesia
- Presurgical
- Acute Chest Syndrome

Simple transfusions are preferred for pediatric patients who suffer a stroke. Exchange transfusion can be used to rapidly reduce the amount of Hgb S. Once a patient has a stroke, they are at risk for additional strokes. Monthly transfusions, either simple or exchange, to maintain HbS concentration below 30% reduces the risk of recurrent stroke. Transfusion of about 10 mL/kg of red blood cells every 3 to 4 weeks is usually sufficient to maintain HbS near 30% and the pretransfusion hematocrit between 25 and 30%.

During transfusion of patients with splenic sequestration, the hemoglobin often increases beyond the expected level, so it is important to transfuse slowly to avoid over-transfusion.

Simple transfusion or exchange transfusion should be considered for patients with refractory priapism. Exchange transfusion has been associated with adverse neurologic sequelae, such as seizures and increased intracranial pressure, so this alternative should be reserved for the most refractory cases.

Patients with sickle cell disease are at high risk for complications during major surgery. Some practitioners recommend that patients be transfused to a hemoglobin of 10 g/dL prior to surgery. Exchange transfusion is not necessary.

Patients with the acute chest syndrome benefit from transfusion early in the course of their disease. Simple transfusion is preferred for patients who are stable. Simple transfusion should only be performed until the hemoglobin reaches about 10 g/dL. Higher levels are associated with vaso-occulsion. Exchange transfusion is recommended for patients who have a rapidly evolving course or do not respond to simple transfusion. There does not appear to be any role for transfusion in the management of routine, uncomplicated painful crises.

Adverse Consequences of Transfusion of Patients with Sickle Cell Disease
Adverse consequences of transfusion of patients with sickle cell disease include alloimmunization, hyperhemolysis and iron overload. Patients with sickle cell disease are chronically transfused and have a high rate of alloimmunization (18-36%). Most patients with sickle cell disease in the United States are African American, and most donors are Caucasian from Western European descent. As a result of this ethnic difference, patients with sickle cell disease are exposed to RBC antigens that they lack, increasing the likelihood of alloantibody formation. The most common antibodies formed in this population are C, E,K1 and Fya . In order to prevent alloimmunization, some centers routinely perform RBC phenotypes on patients with sickle cell disease and only transfuse RBCs that lack C, E,K1 and Fya , if the patient is negative for these antigens. This strategy reduces the rate of antibody formation. A complimentary strategy is to recruit donors who are ethnically similar to sickle cell patients, thereby increasing the likelihood that donors and patients are more antigenically similar.

A serious type of hemolytic transfusion reaction, called the hyperhemolytic syndrome can occur during transfusion of patients with sickle cell disease. In this syndrome, a patient's hemoglobin falls, instead of rises, after transfusion. Both the patient's own RBCs and the transfused RBCs are destroyed even though the transfused RBCs are crossmatch compatible and no new alloantibodies are detectable at the time of transfusion. Further transfusion compounds the problem. Therefore, it is important to recognize this syndrome early and, if possible, discontinue transfusion. If additional transfusions are required because of life-threatening anemia, they should be done cautiously, using concurrent IVIG and steroids.

Each unit of transfused RBCs contains about 200 to 250 mg of iron. With chronic transfusion, iron accumulates in the heart, liver, and endocrine glands. In order to prevent this complication, iron chelating medication is administered. Serum ferritin is serially measured to assess iron stores.

Transfusion Recommendations
Patients with sickle cell disease should not be transfused with RBCs containing Hgb S. Therefore, many laboratories test donor units with a simple solubility test and select units that lack Hgb S. Patients with sickle cell disease should also be transfused with leukocyte reduced blood products to decrease the risk of cytomegalovirus (CMV) transmission, febrile non-hemolytic transfusion reactions, immune suppression, HLA alloimmunization and RBC alloimmunization.

RBCs selected for transfusion of patients with sickle cell disease should be:
- Sickle hemoglobin negative
- Leukoreduced
- Negative for C, E, K[1] and Fy[a] antigens if the patient lacks these antigens
- Negative for any other antigens to which the patient has already been sensitized
- Collected from African American donors if a program exists

NEONATAL ALLOIMMUNE THROMBOCYTOPENIA

Fetomatemal incompatibility for human platelet antigens (HPA) may immunize the mother and cause alloimmune thrombocytopenia in the infant. Most cases are caused by HPA-1a antibody but antibodies to a number of other platelet antigens or, possibly, HLA antibodies are responsible for some cases. Most cases are diagnosed after birth; hence the terminology neonatal alloimmune thrombocytopenia (NAIT). However, the condition develops in utero and the fetus may be severely affected.

The first affected infant is usually unexpected and initial diagnosis is made by exclusion of other causes of neonatal thrombocytopenia. The diagnosis is confirmed by detection of a maternal platelet alloantibody against the father's platelets. Management of subsequent pregnancies concentrates on protecting the fetus from thrombocytopenic bleeding, especially intracranial hemorrhage (ICH).

A major advance is the use of fetal blood sampling for accurate diagnosis and for assessment of the severity of fetal thrombocytopenia. Options for management include maternal treatment with IVIG and/or corticosteroids. For cases considered to be at high risk of ICH, fetal platelet transfusions are the preferred form of management.

After birth the infant is still at risk for intracranial hemorrhage. The platelet count may continue to fall after delivery and the infant's platelets should be counted daily. If there is a perceived risk of bleeding, a platelet transfusion should be given, or high dose IVIG if platelets are not available. Compatible donor platelets or maternal platelets can be used. Maternal platelets should be plasma-reduced or washed with saline.

THROMBOTIC THROMBOCYTOPENIC PURPURA

Thrombotic thrombocytopenic purpura (TTP) and the related disorder, hemolytic uremic syndrome (HUS) are characterized by thrombocytopenia and microangiopathic hemolytic anemia, both resulting from microvascular platelet thrombi in terminal arteries and capillaries. Small vessel occlusion in various organs, notably the brain and kidney, is responsible for the clinical manifestations which include fluctuating neurologic abnormalities and a variable degree of renal insufficiency. On clinical grounds, cases with more of a neurologic presentation have been termed TTP, while those with more pronounced renal involvement often are referred to as HUS. However, clinical overlap is common and some authors use the combined term TTP/HUS.

The classic pentad of findings, consisting of thrombocytopenia, microangiopathic hemolytic anemia, fever, neurologic changes, and renal dysfunction, are seen in only a minority of patients. A high clinical index of suspicion is appropriate because delays in recognition may adversely affect outcomes. Acceptable criteria for a provisional diagnosis include thrombocytopenia and microangiopathic hemolytic anemia in the absence of an alternative cause.

Microangiopathic hemolysis is suggested by the presence of schistocytes on the blood smear. Schistocytes are increased to approximately 4 per field using a 100X oil objective. Neurological symptoms include episodes of focal weakness, visual disturbances, reduced mentation or decreased consciousness, headache, seizure, and coma. Abdominal pain resulting from intestinal and/or pancreatic ischemia may also occur along with nausea, vomiting, and ileus. Even in cases without severe azotemia, renal involvement may be evident, including proteinuria and hematuria.

TTP is classified as primary or secondary depending on whether it occurs on an idiopathic basis or secondary to other medical conditions or treatments.

Primary

- Acute
- Chronic relapsing (familial)

Secondary (Acquired)

- Autoimmune diseases
- Drug-induced - Ticlopidine, clopidogrel, cyclosporine, tacrolimus, quinine and cancer chemotherapy including mitomycin, cis-platinum, gemcitabine, pentostatin
- Cancer
- Transplant-related: allogeneic stem cell transplantation
- Pregnancy/post-partum
- Infection
- Toxin-associated (E. coli 0157:H7, Shigella strains)
- HIV
- Post-operative

Clinical differences have been reported, including faster response to plasma exchange, lower mortality, and higher relapse rates in idiopathic TTP compared with secondary cases.

Considerable evidence now implicates abnormal processing of vonWillebrand Factor (vWF) in the pathogenesis of TTP. The physiological function of vWF is to link platelets with collagen fibers in the subendothelium that is exposed when endothelial cells are injured, thereby promoting clot formation. Under physiologic conditions, von Willebrand Factor (vWF) is released from endothelial cells as circulating ultra-large molecular weight multimers (ULvWF), which have greater adhesive properties and a greater propensity to promote platelet-platelet and platelet-subendothelial interactions. ULvWF are rapidly cleaved by a plasma metalloprotease, called ADAMTS13, (**A D**isintegrin-like **A**nd **M**etalloprotease with **T**hrombo**S**pondin type I motif **13**) into smaller molecular weight multimers.

The presence of ULvWF in many patients with TTP/HUS has been attributed to a deficiency of ADAMTS13. More than 50 mutations in the ADAMTS-13 gene, which result in decreased levels of ADAMTS13, have been detected in patients with familial TTP. The mutations are inherited in an autosomal recessive fashion and only homozygotes or compound heterozygotes with a total absence of protease appear to be affected. Parents of TTP patients, who have ADAMTS13 activity as low as 6 -20% are generally asymptomatic. This data suggests that ADAMTS13 activity as low as 5 -10% is sufficient for prevention of microvascular platelet thrombi.

Decreased vWF cleaving activity has also been detected in patients with idiopathic TTP due to the presence of IgG autoantibody inhibitors. The antibody inhibitors decrease enzyme activity by promoting ADAMTS13 clearance or by interfering with its binding to endothelium. These results have illustrated a common mechanism for the pathogenesis of both familial and acquired TTP and also provided an explanation for the differences in reponse to plasma infusion between these two forms of the disease. Plasma infusion is sufficient to replace deficient enzyme levels in familial TTP cases, but plasma exchange is required to replace enzyme and remove inhibitor in acquired cases.

The value of ADAMTS13 measurements for establishing the diagnosis of TTP and determining the indication for plasma exchange remains uncertain. Although a severe deficiency of ADAMTS13 activity (<5%) in a patient with thrombocytopenia is specific for TTP, it is not predictive of clinical severity. Some patients have the clinical symptoms of TTP with >50%

ADAMTS13 activity, while other individuals have had severe ADAMTS13 deficiency for many years without evidence of illness. Also, patients with TTP and severe ADAMTS13 deficiency are remarkably heterogeneous in their clinical severity. These observations suggest that acquired TTP is not caused by ADAMTS13 deficiency alone and may be triggered by other factors that cause autoimmune reactivity to ADAMTS13 and induce endothelial injury or platelet activation.

Determination of ADAMTS13 activity and inhibitor level is helpful in determining prognosis. Severe ADAMTS13 deficiency identifies a subgroup of patients with a high likelihood of response to plasma exchange. An ADAMTS13 level of <5% predicts an 83% reponse rate, while a level of >5% has a 33% rate. Patients with high titer ADAMTS13 inhibitors require a more prolonged course of plasma exchange and have more complications and high risk of relapse. Specimens for ADAMTS13 activity should be drawn prior to transfusion, because blood components artifactually increase ADAMTS13 activity. The circulating half life of ADAMTS13 is 2.6 days.

Treatment with plasma exchange has reduced mortality in idiopathic TTP from more than 90% to less than 20%. The only randomized controlled clinical trial in TTP was conducted by the Canadian Apheresis Study Group. This study compared plasma infusion (15 ml/kg) with plasma exchange (1.5 plasma volumes per day for 3 days, followed by 1 plasma volume per day). Patients treated with plasma exchange had a survival rate of 78% compared to only 63% for the plasma infusion group. Based in part on the results of this study, plasma exchange has become the standard of care for the management of TTP. Plasma exchange is more beneficial than plasma infusion because it permits delivery of much higher plasma volumes without risk of circulatory overload. Plasma exchange is believed to work by simultaneously replacing deficient ADAMTS-13 enzyme and removing the IgG inhibitor.

Once a diagnosis of TTP has been made, plasma exchange should be initiated as soon as possible. If plasma exchange will be delayed for more than a few hours, plasma should be continuously infused at a dose of 15-30 mL/kg until the procedure is started. Daily plasma exchanges using 40 to 60 mL of ABO compatible plasma per kg of body weight should be performed until the platelet count increases above 150,000/uL. Thereafter, plasma exchange should be performed every other day for at least 5 days after the platelet count and lactate dehydrogenase level have normalized. Often times, 15 to 20 treatments may be necessary to achieve remission. Discontinuing plasma exchange too early may result in relapse. Platelet count, hemoglobin and lactate dehydrogenase (LDH) should be monitored daily throughout the treatment period. LDH level should also be followed closely since it reflects tissue ischemia. However, due to its nonspecificity, near normal levels may be an acceptable endpoint.

Some investigators have advocated using Cryosupernatant instead of FFP because it contains ADAMTS-13 enzyme, but lacks vWF multimers. However, response rates with cryopoor plasma have not been significantly different from FFP.

Although plasma exchange is considered a safe procedure, it should be remembered that serious complications may occur. The University of Oklahoma has reported a major complication rate of 26%. Most of the complications were catheter related and included pulmonary hemorrhage, systemic infection, catheter obstruction, venous thrombosis and hypotension. Two percent of patients have died of complications.

The overall published relapse rate is between 30-40%. A retrospective study conducted by the US TTP Apheresis Study Group found no statistical difference in the rate of relapse when comparing taper to no-taper apheresis schedules. Adjuvant pharmacological therapy may be necessary in refractory cases. Since the discovery of the autoimmune basis of idiopathic TTP, there has been renewed interest in the use of immunosuppressive therapy. The role of glucocorticoids remains unclear with comparable mortality rates reported in the literature. If not used initially, they are frequently added later if response to plasma exchange is delayed. Another immunosuppressive approach involves the anti-CD20 monoclonal antibody, Rituximab. The time until remission averages 2 to 5 weeks. Splenectomy has also proven successful in preventing relapses, reducing the attack rate from 2.3 +/- 2 events per year to 0.1 +/- .1 events per year.

Antiplatelet agents have not proved to be particularly beneficial in the treatment of TTP and may increase the risk of hemorrhage, particularly with severe thrombocytopenia. Both ticlopidine and clopidogrel have been associated with induction of autoantibodies to ADAMTS-13, resulting in drug-induced TTP and should not be used as therapy.

HEPARIN INDUCED THROMBOCYOPENIA

Heparin induced thrombocytopenia (HIT) is the most significant adverse effect of heparin therapy after bleeding. Two categories of HIT are recognized; a benign form called type I and an immune mediated form associated with thrombosis called type II. Type I HIT is caused be a direct interaction of heparin with platelets. Type II HIT is caused by an antibody directed against heparin-PF4 (platelet factor 4) complexes, which bind to and activate platelets, leading to thrombocytopenia and thrombosis. The interaction of this immune complex with platelet membranes activates platelets, releases additional platelet factor 4, and perpetuates the cycle of platelet activation, thrombocytopenia, and thrombosis.

Type I HIT affects up to 10% of patients treated with heparin. Platelet counts decrease rapidly within the first two days of heparin exposure, but usually remain above 100,000/uL. Platelet counts return to normal within two days in spite of continued heparin therapy. This type of HIT is not associated with an increased risk of thrombosis or any other adverse clinical consequences. No intervention is necessary.

The incidence of type II HIT is 2.6% of patients exposed to unfractionated heparin and 0.2% exposed to low molecular weight heparin. Approximately 25% of these patients will develop thrombosis within 30 days. Most cases arise in patients who have not been previously exposed to heparin. In this situation, thrombocytopenia usually occurs 5 to 12 days after heparin initiation. In patients who have been previously sensitized to heparin, platelet counts may decrease within the first three days or even hours after re-exposure. Platelet counts usually decrease more than 50% from baseline and typically fall to 20,000 - 100,000/ uL. The nadir is usually reached 5 days after onset of the decline. After discontinuing heparin, platelet counts begin to rise within 2-3 days and usually return to normal within 10 days. Antibody decreases to undetectable levels within 2-3 months after cessation of heparin therapy. Future exposure to heparin is contraindicated.

The thrombosis associated with type II HIT usually involves major vessels, particularly the distal aorta and femoral arteries. Numerous complications have been reported including stroke, pulmonary embolism, myocardial infarction, mural thrombosis, mesenteric infarction, renal infarction, adrenal infarction, and distal limb gangrene. Patients with preexisting cardiovascular disease or recent cardiovascular surgery are prone to arterial thrombosis, while other postoperative patients are more likely to experience venous thrombosis.

Any heparin compound can induce antibody formation, but those forms with the highest molecular weight and highest degree of sulfation are associated with the highest incidence of HIT type II. The types of heparin reported to cause HIT II in order of decreasing frequency are bovine heparin> porcine heparin> low molecular weight heparin> heparinoids. Low molecular weight heparin appears to induce antibody formation about one fourth as often as bovine heparin and seldom causes thrombocytopenia. HIT can be induced by any dose or route of heparin administration, including heparin flushes and heparin coated intra-arterial lines. High dose IV heparin is more likely to induce antibody formation than low dose subcutaneous heparin. Long duration of heparin administration is more likely to cause HIT, but the syndrome can occur after a single bolus.

Heparin should be discontinued in any patient with a clinical presentation consistent with HIT type II. Heparin flushes and heparin coated catheters should also be avoided. Platelet transfusions are contraindicated because they may contribute to thrombus formation or extension. If continued anticoagulation is required, Coumadin should be initiated as soon as the platelet count begins to recover. Low molecular weight heparin should not be used, because antibody cross-reacts with it in 90% of cases. Heparinoids react with HIT antibody in 7 to 20% of cases. Elective procedures requiring heparin therapy should be delayed until antibody is no longer detectable. If a patient with a history of HIT type II needs to undergo open heart surgery, they should be retested for heparin antibody. If the test is negative, they can be exposed to heparin during bypass and then switched to a direct thrombin inhibitor postoperatively.

Patients receiving heparin should have a platelet count performed at least once every three days. If HIT type II is suspected, the diagnosis can be confirmed by laboratory tests that detect the antibody. An ELISA method is used for heparin antibody detection that has a sensitivity of 90% and a specificity of 98% for diagnosis of HIT.

DRUG INDUCED THROMBOCYTOPENIA

Drug induced thrombocytopenia can be caused by dozens of different medications and should be suspected in any patient who presents with acute thrombocytopenia of unknown origin. Typically, a patient will have taken the sensitizing drug for about 1 week or intermittently over a longer period of time before presenting with petechial hemorrhages and ecchymoses. Platelet inhibitors are the exception to this general rule because petechiae may occur within 1 or 2 days after an apparent first exposure. Systemic symptoms such as lightheadedness, chills, fever, nausea, and vomiting often precede bleeding. Severely affected individuals have florid purpura and bleeding from nose, gums and gastrointestinal or urinary tract. In adults, the presence of severe thrombocytopenia, with a platelet count <20,000/uL, increases the likelihood that a patient has drug induced thrombocytopenia. If the causative medication is promptly discontinued, symptoms often resolve within 2 days and the platelet count returns to normal within a week.

The medications most commonly associated with drug induced thrombocytopenia are listed below.

Analgesics
- Acetaminophen
- Diclofenac
- Ibuprofen
- Naproxen
- Propoxyphene

Anticonvulsant & sedatives
- Carbamazepine
- Diazepam
- Fentanyl
- Phenytoin
- Trimipramine
- Valproic acid

Antimicrobial
- Cephalosporins
- Linezolid
- Penicillins
- Rifampin
- Sulfonamides
- Trimethoprim
- Vancomycin

Cardiac
- Amrinone
- Beta blockers
- Digoxin
- Procainamide

Chemotherapeutic
- Fludarabine
- Oxaliplatin

Cinchona alkaloids
- Quinine
- Quinidine

Diuretics
- Chlorothiazide
- Furosemide
- Hydrochlorothiazide

Heparins
- Unfractionated
- Low molecular weight

Histamine Receptor Antagonists
- Cimetidine
- Ranitidine

Immune Modulators
- Cyclosporine
- Interferon alpha & beta
- Rituximab

Platelet Inhibitors
- Abciximab
- Clopidogrel
- Dipyridamole
- Eptifibatide
- Tirofiban

Rheumatic

- D-penicillamine
- Gold salts
- Infliximab

Many cases of drug induced thrombocytopenia are immune mediated and it is often possible to identify antibodies that react with normal platelets in the presence of the drug but not in its absence. In other cases with a high index of suspicion for drug induced thrombocytopenia, antibody tests are negative, probably because a drug metabolite produced in vivo, rather than the parent drug, is the sensitizing agent. Testing for drug induced platelet antibodies, with the exception of heparin, is technically demanding and only available at a few reference laboratories. Therefore, it is not useful in the immediate care of a patient.

When there is uncertainty about the causative drug, all medications should be discontinued, and pharmacologic equivalents with different chemical structures substituted as necessary. Patients who present with severe thrombocytopenia and wet purpura should be treated with platelet transfusions because of the risk of fatal intracranial and intrapulmonary hemorrhage. The therapeutic benefit of corticosteroids and intravenous immune globulin has not been proven. Once established, drug sensitivity probably persists indefinitely and patients should be advised to avoid permanently the suspected medication.

XIGRIS THERAPY

Xigris (drotrecogin alfa) is a recombinant form of human activated Protein C that is used in the treatment of severe sepsis. Activated Protein C exerts an antithrombotic effect by inhibiting coagulation factors Va and VIIIa and has an indirect profibrinolytic activity through its ability to inhibit plasminogen activator inhibitor-1 (PAI-1). Xigris variably prolongs the aPTT, but has minimal effect on the PT.

Bleeding is the most common adverse effect associated with Xigris therapy. The risk of serious bleeding increases if the patient has thrombocytopenia or has recently been treated with oral anticoagulants, heparin, glycoprotein IIb/IIIa inhibitors, aspirin, or clopidogrel. If bleeding occurs, the infusion of Xigris should immediately be stopped. In the majority of patients, plasma concentrations fall below detectable levels (10 ng/mL) within 2 hours after stopping infusion. In the event of serious hemorrhaging, transfusion of FFP and cryoprecipitate may be necessary.

CHAPTER 10:
Transfusion Therapy for ABO Mismatched Allogenic Blood & Marrow Transplant Patients

The inheritance of ABO blood group antigens is independent of HLA antigens, so an HLA-matched donor is commonly of a blood group different from that of the recipient. Red cell incompatibility does not preclude allogeneic transplantation because blood group antigens are not major histocompatibility antigens and stem cells do not express blood group antigens. However, appropriate measures must be taken to avoid acute or delayed hemolytic reactions during transplantation involving either minor or major incompatibility.

MINOR ABO INCOMPATIBILITY

The transplant may involve a minor ABO incompatibility in which the donor possesses anti-A and/or anti-B capable of reacting with A and/or B antigens on the recipient's red cells and tissues. The most common examples involve a group O donor marrow being transplanted to a group A, B, or AB recipient.

Minor ABO mismatched transplant prior to high dose chemotherapy
Blood components that contain large volumes of plasma, such as platelets and FFP, should be of the recipient's blood type to avoid infusion of incompatible anti-A and/or anti-B that may hemolyze recipient RBCs or delay engraftment. RBC units should also be of the recipient's ABO group up to the beginning of high dose chemotherapy.

Minor ABO mismatched transplant after high dose chemotherapy
Once high dose chemotherapy is administered, no new red blood cells of the recipient's type will be made by the patient's bone marrow, but circulating recipient RBCs will persist for several months because the average life span of RBCs is 120 days. Therefore, one should continue to transfuse platelets of the recipient's ABO group, to avoid giving large volumes of incompatible anti-A and anti-B, until the patient's original RBCs are no longer detected.

A delayed hemolytic reaction resulting from the transient production of anti-A and anti-B by donor lymphocytes infused with the marrow may occur between 7 and 14 days after transplantation. RBC transfusions should be of the donor's ABO group to avoid any possibility of hemolysis.

Minor ABO mismatched Marrow or Peripheral Blood Stem Cell Product
Marrow or stem cell collections involving minor ABO mismatches may be plasma depleted to remove as much anti-A and/or anti-B as possible. This modification minimizes the possibility of an immediate hemolytic reaction during marrow or stem cell infusion.

MAJOR ABO INCOMPATIBILITY

A transplant with a major ABO incompatibility occurs when the recipient possesses anti-A and/or anti-B capable of reacting with ABO antigens on donor red cells. The most common examples involve a group A, B, or AB donor begin transplanted to a group O recipient.

Major ABO mismatched transplant prior to high dose chemotherapy
Both RBCs and blood components that contain large volumes of plasma, such as platelets and FFP, should be of the recipient's blood type up until the beginning of high dose chemotherapy.

Major ABO mismatched transplant after high dose chemotherapy
Recipient anti-A and/or anti-B may persist for several months after high dose chemotherapy and transplantation. Therefore, only RBCs of the recipient's ABO group should be transfused as long as anti-A and/or anti-B are detectable. Platelets and FFP should be switched to the donor's ABO type to avoid transfusion of large volumes of incompatible anti-A and/or anti-B that would destroy RBCs of the donor type.

Major ABO mismatched Marrow or Peripheral Blood Stem Cell Product
Bone marrows involving major ABO mismatches undergo RBC depletion to remove as many incompatible RBCs as possible. This modification minimizes the possibility of an immediate hemolytic reaction during marrow infusion. Major ABO mismatches are often associated with delayed erythropoiesis, requiring more transfusion support than ABO compatible transplants.

MINOR & MAJOR ABO INCOMPATIBILITIES

In some instances, both major and minor incompatibilities exist simultaneously, such as a transplant involving a group B donor and a group A recipient or vice versa.

Minor & major ABO mismatched transplant prior to high dose chemotherapy
Both platelets and RBCs should be of the recipient's ABO group.

Minor & major ABO mismatched transplant after high dose chemotherapy
Group O RBCs should be issued until the patient's original anti-A or anti-B is no longer detected. Thereafter, RBCs of the donor's ABO group can be issued. Group AB platelets and FFP should be issued because they are devoid of anti-A and anti-B and will not hemolyze the recipient's circulating RBCs or new donor RBCs being released from the marrow following engraftment. Once the recipient's original RBCs are no longer detectable, platelets and FFP should be switched to the donor's ABO group.

ABO Incompatibility		Blood Components	Up to Start of Preparative Regimen	Start of Preparative Regimen	Stem Cell Infusion	Original Antibody Undetectable	Original RBCs Undetectable
MAJOR Recip	Donor						
O	A	RBC's	O	O	O	A	Not Applicable
		Plts/Plasma	O	A (AB)	A (AB)	A	
O	B	RBC's	O	O	O	B	Not Applicable
		Plts/Plasma	O	B (BA)	B (BA)	B	
A	AB	RBC's	A	A	A	AB	Not Applicable
		Plts/Plasma	A	AB (A, B)	AB (A, B)	AB	
B	AB	RBC's	B	B	B	AB	Not Applicable
		Plts/Plasma	B	AB (B, A)	AB (B, A)	AB	
O	AB	RBC's	O	O	O	AB	Not Applicable
		Plts/Plasma	O	AB (A, B)	AB (A, B)	AB	
MINOR Recip	Donor						
A	O	RBC's	A	O	O	Not Applicable	O
		Plts/Plasma	A	A (AB)	A (AB)		O
B	O	RBC's	B	O	O	Not Applicable	O
		Plts/Plasma	B	B (BA)	B (AB)		O
AB	O	RBC's	AB	O	O	Not Applicable	O
		Plts/Plasma	AB	AB (A, B)	AB (A, B)		O
AB	A	RBC's	AB	A	A	Not Applicable	A
		Plts/Plasma	AB	AB (A, B)	AB (A, B)		A
AB	B	RBC's	AB	B	B	Not Applicable	B
		Plts/Plasma	AB	AB (B, A)	AB (B, A)		B
MAJOR & MINOR Recip	Donor						
A	B	RBC's	A	O	O	B	B
		Plts/Plasma	A	AB (A, B)	AB (A, B)	AB (A, B)	B
B	A	RBC's	B	O	O	A	A
		Plts/Plasma	B	AB (B, A)	AB (A, B)	AB (B, A)	A
RH Incompatibility		Blood Components	Up to Start of Preparative Regimen	Start of Preparative Regimen	Stem Cell Infusion	D Antigen Undetectable	D Antigen Detectable
Recip	Donor						
Rh pos	Rh neg	RBC's	Pos	Neg	Neg	Neg	Neg
		Plts/Plasma	Pos or Neg	Pos or Neg	Pos or Neg	Pos or Neg	Pos or Neg
Rh neg	Rh pos	RBC's	Neg	Neg	Neg	Neg	Pos
		Plts/Plasma	Pos or Neg	Pos or Neg	Pos or Neg	Pos or Neg	Pos or Neg

( ) indicates 2nd, then 3rd choices for platelets

Apheresis platelets are preferred over random donor platelets; if the first choice blood type in apheresis platelets is not available, use random platelets before going to apheresis platelets of the second choice blood type. Up to start of Preparative Regimen (high dose chemotherapy) and after they have converted to donor type, platelet transfusions should follow usual protocols for blood type.

HEMOLYSIS FOLLOWING ALLOGENEIC BMT

Minor incompatibility (e.g. group O donor marrow infused to group A recipient)

An important complication of minor ABO-incompatible marrow transplants is known as the passenger lymphocyte syndrome. Immune hemolysis of the recipient's red cells occurs as a result of anti-A and/or anti-B production by passenger lymphocytes in the marrow product.

Rarely, antibodies of other blood group systems, particularly Rh, may also cause hemolysis. Hemolysis occurs suddenly between days 5 & 15 after transplant, before engraftment & immune reconstitution. Patients experience intravascular hemolysis, rapidly decreasing hemoglobin & renal failure. Anti-A &/or B directed against recipient RBCs is detected in serum and on RBCs. Hemolysis subsides as patient's residual incompatible RBCs are destroyed and replaced by new RBCs of donor origin and/or transfused group O RBCs. At risk patients need to be monitored between days 5 and 15 after transplant by measuring hemoglobin, bilirubin, lactate dehydrogenase, haptoglobin and direct antiglobulin test. It is very important to avoid transfusion of platelets with ABO incompatible plasma. If hemolysis occurs, appropriate management consists of transfusion of group O red cells. Occasionally a red cell exchange transfusion is indicated to replace the recipient's incompatible red cells with those that are group O.

Major incompatibility (e.g. group A donor marrow infused to group O recipient)

The recipient is capable of making antibodies against donor's RBC antigens. Most cases are prevented by RBC depletion of the marrow before infusion. Delayed hemolysis may occur when there is persistence of recipient's anti-A &/or B. Hemolysis occurs more often in patients being treated with cyclosporine. Hemolysis begins between days 35 & 105 after transplant and can persist for 10 to 100 days. High titer anti-A and/or B inhibit erythropoiesis & may cause RBC aplasia. As anti-A &/or B titer decreases, erythropoiesis occurs but RBCs are hemolyzed by the persistent antibody. Hemolysis resolves with disappearance of patient's anti-A &/or B. At risk patients need to be monitored between days 35 & 105 for hemoglobin, bilirubin, LD, haptoglobin and DAT.

Autoimmune Hemolytic Anemia

Autoimmune hemolytic anemia (AIHA) has occurred with matched sibling & matched unrelated donors. It may occur more commonly with T cell depleted marrow grafts. Hemolysis is due to antibodies produced by donor's lymphocytes against RBCs of donor origin. It usually begins 7 to 25 months after transplant and is often resistant to therapy. Patients need to be monitored after the 7th month for hemoglobin, bilirubin, lactate dehydrogenase, haptoglobin and direct antiglobulin test.

Thrombotic Thrombocytopenic Purpura

TTP is associated with total body irradiation, chemotherapeutic & immunosuppressive drugs, and bone marrow or solid organ transplant. TTP usually develops at a median of 5 months (range 3 – 7 months) after transplant. Lack of RBC antibodies and presence of fragmented RBCs on peripheral smear help to distinguish TTP from immune hemolysis.

Passive Transfer of Antibody

The most common sources are plasma of donor marrow, platelet transfusions & intravenous immunoglobulin.Hemolysis occurs immediately after infusion of large volumes of these products.

CHAPTER 11:
Management of Hemophilia and von Willebrand's Disease

Coagulation factor concentrates may be prepared either from large volumes of pooled normal plasma or cryoprecipitate by various separation methods that are treated for virus inactivation or by recombinant DNA technology. In spite of the safeguards, plasma derived factor concentrates still carry a slight risk of viral or prion transmission. Recombinant factor concentrates are considered to be safer.

The concentrates are supplied in lyophilized form and the quantity of the coagulation factor activity is stated on the label. Ideally, the medical director of the transfusion service should be involved in the treatment of coagulation factor deficiencies, helping to determine the product of choice and the dosage.

HEMOPHILIA A

Hemophilia A is a bleeding disorder caused by Factor VIII deficiency. Characteristic laboratory findings include prolonged aPTT, normal protime, and normal fibrinogen. The prolonged aPTT is due to the Factor VIII deficiency. One unit of Factor VIII activity is defined as the Factor VIII content of 1 mL of fresh, citrated, pooled, normal plasma. Disease severity correlates with factor VIII activity. Patients with factor VIII levels less than 1% are classified as severe, 1-5% as moderate and >5% as mild hemophilia A.

Treatment Guidelines
Desmopressin (1-deamino-8-d-arginine vasopressin, DDAVP) results in a transient fourfold increase in plasma Factor VIII levels by stimulating the release of Factor VIII and vonWillebrand's factor from storage sites. Most mild hemophiliacs with factor VIII levels greater than 8% will respond to DDAVP. Therefore, it provides an alternative therapy for minor bleeding in most patients with mild hemophilia A. DDAVP is administered either intranasally or intravenously.. Repeat doses can be given at 12 to 24 hour intervals, but 2-3 consecutive daily doses may cause side effects.

Patients with moderate or severe hemophilia A usually require treatment with Factor VIII concentrate. The patient's Factor VIII level should be measured prior to the loading dose to calculate dosage and after the loading dose to determine adequacy of the dose. Trough levels should be measured prior to each maintenance dose. Doses are usually scheduled at 12- hour intervals because the circulating half-life of Factor VIII is 8 to 12 hours. One unit of infused Factor VIII should raise the plasma level by approximately 2%. The following formula is used to calculate Factor VIII dosage:

$$\# \text{ Factor VIII Units} = \frac{wt(kg) \times desired \% \text{ increase}}{2}$$

When bleeding is severe, the appropriate loading dose of Factor VIII concentrate is 50 units/kg, which should result in a factor level of 80 –100%. Control of serious bleeding requires hospitalization and factor VIII boluses every 8 to 12 hours to maintain trough levels above 50%. A plasma level of 30-50% is usually sufficient for less severe bleeding. One to three doses are usually sufficient to control mild bleeding, prevent secondary hemorrhage, and initiate tissue healing.The following general treatment recommendations are for individuals without Factor VIII inhibitors.

Factor VIII Dosing Recommendations

Bleeding Site	Loading Dose Units/Kg	Desired Plasma FVIII Level %	Maintenance Dose - Units/Kg
Oral mucosa	20	30 - 50	20 q 12 hours
Epistaxis	40 - 50	80 - 100 initial, then 30	30 - 40
Joint	20 - 40	30 - 50	20 q 12 hours
Muscle	20 - 30	>50	20 q 12 hours
CSN	50	100 initial, then 50 - 100	25 q 12 hours
Abdominal pain	20 - 40	>50	20 - 40 q 12 hours
Gastrointestinal	40 - 50	100 intial, then 30	30 - 40 q 12 hours
Genitourinary	40 - 50	100 intial, then 30	30 - 40 q 12 hours
Neck hemorrhage	50	100	25 - 30 q 12 hours
Major trauma	50	100 intial, then 50	25 - 30 q 12 hours
Surgery prophylaxis	50	100 intial, then 50	25 - 30 q 12 hours
Dental procedure	20	30 - 50	20 q 12 hours

Inhibitors to Factor VIII

Approximately 20-30% of patients with severe hemophilia A develop antibodies to Factor VIII that neutralize or inhibit coagulant activity, making replacement therapy ineffective. These antibodies are referred to as inhibitors and occur almost exclusively in patients with severe hemophilia A. The presence of an inhibitor does not increase the frequency of bleeding, but does increase morbidity and mortality, including less well controlled hemorrhage, more joint damage, and increased hospitalization. The strength of an inhibitor is measured with the Bethesda assay which determines the dilution of patient plasma that decreases normal plasma Factor VIII activity by 50%. The result is expressed as Bethesda units and classified as low (<10 BU), intermediate (10-20 BU), and high (>20 BU) titers.

Treatment of Patients with Inhibitors

Treatment of bleeding in patients with inhibitors is challenging. One reatment strategy involves bypassing Factor VIII in the coagulation cascade. Recombinant Factor VIIa (NovoSeven) received FDA approval and became commercially available in 1999. NovoSeven is indicated for the treatment of bleeding episodes in hemophilia A or B patients with inhibitors to Factor VIII or Factor IX. Recombinant Factor VIIa is supplied in three sizes: 1200 μg/vial, 2400 μg/vial and 4800 μg/vial The recommended dose is 90 μg/kg by IV bolus given every two hours for 24 hours or until hemostasis is achieved. Once the patient is stabilized, the interval between treatments can be lengthened to 3-6 hours. This dosage schedule can be used for patients undergoing major surgery or treatment of serious CNS, intraperitoneal, retroperitoneal, or intramuscular bleeding. The goal of therapy should be to increase peak levels of FVII functional clotting activity (FVII: C) measured immediately after the initial dose, to above 30% and preferably between 60 and 90 %. The protime shortens significantly and often plateaus around 7 seconds; the aPTT may shorten as much as 15 to 20, but usually does not completely normalize.

Acquired Hemophilia A

Autoantibodies to Factor VIII occasionally develop in healthy elderly adults, postpartum women, and patients with autoimmune disease or cancer; the majority of cases, however, have no known etiology. Patients with acquired factor VIII deficiency are at risk for spontaneous intramuscular hematomas, soft tissue hemorrhage, and mucosal bleeding. Spontaneous remission occurs in 30-40% of patients. Elective surgical procedures should be postponed while the patient is observed for possible spontaneous remission. Treatment options include:

Recombinant Factor VIIa, recombinant Factor VIII, DDAVP, intravenous immunoglobulin, and immunosuppressive drugs. DDAVP should be more successful in acquired hemophilia since these patients can synthesize Factor VIII. Patients with autoantibodies do not usually mount an anamnestic response to Factor VIII infusion. Dosage is calculated as for congenital inhibitors.

HEMOPHILIA B (FACTOR IX DEFICIENCY)

Hemophilia B (Factor IX deficiency, Christmas disease) causes a prolonged aPTT in the presence of a normal protime. Severity of disease is classified according to the Factor IX level. Patients with Factor IX levels <1% are classified as severe, 1-5% as moderate and 6-60% as mild hemophila B.

Treatment Guidelines
The treatment of choice for Factor IX deficiency is recombinant Factor IX. A specimen for Factor IX level should be drawn before the loading dose to determine the baseline level, 1 hour after the dose to determine the peak level, and immediately before the next dose to determine the trough level. Caution must be exercised in calculating the dosage of recombinant Factor IX. For example, BeneFIX has lower recovery values than plasma derived Factor IX concentrate due to differences in the post-translational modification of the final protein. In some cases the observed rise in Factor IX level may only be 50% of the expected value. Therefore, higher doses of BeneFIX may be required. The BeneFIX package insert recommends the following dosage calculation:

#Factor IX units required = Body weight (kg) X desired Factor IX increase (%) X 1.2

However, because of the wide variation in recovery between individuals a factor greater than 1.2 may be necessary.

When bleeding is severe, the appropriate dose of Factor IX is 100-120 units/kg, which should result in a factor IX level of 80-100%. General dosage guidelines are summarized in the following table.

Factor IX Dosing Recommendations

Bleeding Site	Loading Dose Units/Kg	Desired Plasma FVIII Level %	Maintenance Dose - Units/Kg
Oral mucosa	50	30 - 50	Usually not required
Epistaxis	80 - 100	80 - 100 initial, then 30	70 - 80 qod
Joint	30 - 40	30 - 50	30 - 40 qod as needed
Muscle	40 - 60	>50	40 - 60 qod
CSN	100	100 initial, then 50 - 100	50 q 24 hours
Gastrointestinal	80 - 100	100 intial, then 30	70 - 80 qod
Genitourinary	80 - 100	100 intial, then 30	70 - 80 qod
Major trauma	100	100 intial, then 50	100 q 24 hours
Surgery prophylaxis	50	100 intial, then 50	100 q 24 hours

Factor IX Inhibitors
Inhibitors develop in only 1 to 4% of persons with hemophilia B. Approximately 40% have titers less than 5 BU, while the majority has higher titers. Patients with low titers (< 10 Bethesda units) can be treated with sufficient quantities of Factor IX concentrate to overwhelm the inhibitor. Some patients with inhibitors to Factor IX have severe allergic reactions when treated with any plasma product containing Factor IX. Recombinant Factor VIIa is

recommended for these patients and for any patient with a high titer inhibitor. The recommended dose is 90 $\mu g/kg$ by IV bolus given every two hours until hemostasis is achieved. For severe bleeds, dosing should be continued at 3 to 6 hour intervals to maintain hemostasis.

VON WILLEBRAND'S DISEASE

Von Willebrand's disease (vWD) is the most common inherited abnormality of hemostasis and is usually inherited in an autosomal dominant fashion. Currently, vWD is divided into 3 types (type 1,2 and 3) and type 2 vWD is further divided into 4 subclasses (2A, 2B, 2M, and 2N). Estimates of prevalence vary from 1 per 10,000 persons to 1 per 100 persons, with Type 1 vWD being the most common type.

von Willebrand's Disease Characteristics

vWD Type	Prevalence	Inheritance	vWF Defect
Type 1	70% vWD cases	Autosomal Dominant	Partial quantitative vWF deficiency
Type 2	25% vWD cases		Qualitative vWF abnormalities
Type 2A	75% Type 2 cases	Autosomal Dominant	
Type 2B	20% Type 2 cases	Autosomal Dominant	vWF increased affinity for platelets
Type 2M	<5% Type 2 cases	Autosomal Dominant	Functional defect in multimers
Type 2N	<5% Type 2 cases	Autosomal Recessive	Decreased FVIII binding
Type 3	<10% vWD cases	Autosomal Recessive	Quantitative vWF deficiency

VWD is due to a qualitative or quantitative abnormality of von Willebrand factor (vWF), leading to a disruption of primary hemostasis. Normally, vWF mediates the adhesion and aggregation of platelets to subendothelium in blood vessels with high shear force, such as arteries. In addition, vWF binds to factor VIIIc and protects it against degradation. Substantial deficiency of vWF (levels <30%) results in a primary hemostatic defect and most patients present with mild mucocutaneous bleeding including easy bruising, epistaxis, posttraumatic and postsurgical bleeding and menorrhagia in women. Cases of Type 3 vWD with very low vWF also have very low factor VIII levels and may experience soft tissue and joint hemorrhages.

A panel of tests is required to screen adequately for the disorder, because routine screening tests such as the aPTT may be normal. The aPTT is abnormal only in those cases of vWD with low levels of factor VIIIc. The initial panel includes factor VIIIc assay, von Willebrand factor antigen, and ristocetin cofactor (RcoF). VWF antigen test measures the quantity of vWF in plasma. RcoF assesses vWF function by measuring the binding activity of vWF to platelet glycoprotein 1b. Patient plasma is added to fixed donor platelets, ristocetin is added, and the rate of platelet aggregation is measured. Ristocetin is a small glycopeptide antibiotic that binds to both vWF and GP1b, resulting in a vWF dependent platelet agglutination. Factor VIII coagulant activity provides information about the ability of vWF to function as a carrier protein for factor VIII. Factor VIII is always decreased in patients with Type 2N and Type 3 vWD. Factor VIII coagulant activity does not always parallel vWF antigen levels.

If one or more of the initial tests are abnormal, additional testing may performed to further classify vWD. Ristocetin induced platelet aggregation (RIPA) is particularly useful to distinguish ttype 2A from type 2B vWD, because it can demonstrate the higher than normal affinity of vWF for the platelet GP1b/IX complex that occurs in Type 2a. In this assay, varying concentrations of ristocetin (0.5, 1.0, & 1.5 mg/mL) are mixed together with platelet rich plasma. The minimal concentration of ristocetin able to cause 30% platelet aggregation is recorded. Platelets from unaffected individuals require 1.0 – 1.5 mg/dL of ristocetin for aggregation. Platelets from patients with type 2A will not aggregate with 0.5 mg/mL ristocetin, but platelets from patients with type 2B do.

VWF multimer analysis involves the separation of vWF molecules by protein electrophoresis and detection of all molecular weight forms by Western Blot. This test is used to subclassify Type 2 vWD into types 2A, 2B and 2M. Types 2A and 2B have a decrease in high molecular weight multimers, while type 2M has a normal distribution.

Based on the levels of RcoF, vWF antigen, factor VIII activity and distribution of vWF multimers, vWD can be classified into quantitative (Types 1 & 3) and qualitative (Type 2) abnormalities. Quantitative abnormalities include a mild to moderate reduction of vWF (Type 1) or complete absence of vWF (Type 3). In contrast, Type 2A & 2B vWD have a normal quantity of vWF, which is functionally and structurally defective as manifested by a discordant decrease in RcoF activity. Panel results are interpreted as follows:

Classification of von Willebrand's Disease

vWD Type	RcoF	vWF Ag	FVIIIc	Platelet count	Low Dose RIPA	Multimers
1	Decreased	Decreased	Normal / Decreased	Normal	Absent	All MW decreased
2A	Decreased	Normal / Borderline	Normal / Decreased	Normal	Absent	High MW decreased
2B	Decreased	Normal / Borderline	Normal / Decreased	Decreased	Present	High MW decreased
2M	Decreased	Normal / Decreased	Normal	Normal	Absent	Normal
2N	Normal	Normal	Decreased	Normal	Absent	Normal
3	Absent	Absent	Marked Decreased	Normal	Absent	Absent

Type I vWD is the mildest form of the disease and is characterized by a concordant mild quantitative decrease in vWF level and ristocetin cofactor activity (30-50%). Factor VIIIc may be normal or decreased.

Type 2 vWD is caused by a qualitative defect in vWF that may be associated with deficient multimerization. VWF antigen level and RcoF activities are often discordant; Rcof is usually low and vWF and FVIII are usually borderline. Type 2 vWD can be further subclassified into as type 2A, 2B, 2M, or 2N.

- Type 2A is a qualitative variant of vWF characterized by absence of high molecular weight multimers. The absence of these high molecular weight multimers results in decreased RcoF activity. Factor VIIIc activity may be normal to moderately reduced. Platelet rich plasma from patients with Type 2A do not aggregate in the presence of dilute ristocetin.
- Type 2B vWD is characterized by a dysfunctional vWF that has increased platelet avidity, resulting in increased platelet aggregation with dilute ristocetin. Patients with Type 2B often have mild thrombocytopenia. Platelet rich plasma from patients with Type 2B does aggregate with dilute ristocetin.
- Type 2M (M for multimers) has a normal vWF multimer distribution, but the binding of vWF to platelets is decreased.
- Type 2N (N for Normandy) resembles hemophilia A in that plasma factor VIIIc levels are decreased. A defect in binding of vWF to Factor VIII results in increased clearance of Factor VIIIc.

Type III vWD is the most severe form of vWD. There is almost total absence of vWF in the plasma and platelets and markedly decreased factor VIIIc.

Mild vWD may be difficult to detect because assay values in a patient may vary at different times. Repeat testing after an interval of 2 to 4 weeks may be required to confirm or exclude the diagnosis. Inflammation, stress, pregnancy or estrogen therapy may increase vWF levels above baseline and potentially mask diagnosis of mild vWD. Short term physical exertion causes a rapid increase in vWF levels. Combined oral contraceptive pills increase vWF levels. Repeat testing should be undertaken 4 to 6 weeks after discontinuation of oral contraceptives. Hyperthyroidism increases vWF levels and hypothyroidism is associated with decreased levels. People with blood group O have 25% lower vWF levels than patients with non-O blood groups.

Myeloproliferative disorders and monoclonal gammopathies are associated with acquired abnormalities of vWF, often due to immune clearance. The high shear stress associated with aortic stenosis causes proteolysis of high molecular weight multimers and mimics type 2 vWD.

Treatment Options
Treatment of vWD can be accomplished by stimulating the release of endogenously stored vWF or infusing exogenous vWF.

Treatment Recommendations for vWD

vWD Type	Minor - Moderate Bleeding	Major Bleeding
Type 1	DDAVP & antifibrinolytic	Factor Concentrate
Type 2A	DDAVP & antifibrinolytic	Factor Concentrate
Type 2B	Factor Concentrate	Factor Concentrate
Type 3	Factor Concentrate	Factor Concentrate

DDAVP promotes accelerated release of endogenous vWF from storage sites and is the treatment of choice for Type 1 vWD. It can be used prophylactically prior to surgery and to treat bleeding. Type 1 vWD patients with baseline plasma levels of vWF antigen in the 10 to 20 IU/dL range or higher are those who are more likely to reach post-DDAVP levels sufficient to attain hemostasis. DDAVP is usually ineffective for Type 2 variants and Type 3. It can cause thrombocytopenia in Type 2B patients. A therapeutic trial of DDAVP before an elective procedure is advisable. Factor VIII and vWF are measured before and 1, 4 and 8 hours after infusion. Responsive patients have will have a three-fold increase in Factor VIII:C and a two-fold increase in vWF within 30 minutes. Increased levels should persist for 8 to 10 hours. Baseline and post-infusion platelet counts should be measured in unclassified patients to screen for thrombocytopenia. If the trial is successful, the same dose can be used for prophylaxis or treatment of bleeding. Doses should be repeated on a daily basis for most bleeding episodes. Tachyphylaxis may occur with more frequent dosing or after 3 to 4 consecutive days. It can be overcome by waiting 24 to 48 hours before giving the next dose. Side effects include flushing, headache, hyponatremia, and hypotension. Hypotension is most often associated with rapid infusion. It is especially important to monitor Infants and surgical patients for hyponatremia.

Antifibrinolytic amino acids, such as epsilon aminocaproic acid (Amicar) are often prescribed as an adjunct to desmopressin therapy when treating epistaxis, oral cavity bleeding, bleeding associated with dental procedures, and menorrhagia. Amicar interferes with the lysis of newly formed clots by saturating the binding sites on plasminogen and preventing its attachment to fibrin.

Factor Replacement Therapy for vWD

Factor replacement is recommended for patients with Types 2 and 3 vWD and for Type 1 patients who do not respond adequately to DDAVP. The FDA has licensed some Factor VIII concentrates containing multimeric vWF, such as Humate P and Koate-DVI, for treatment of vWD.

Humate P is labeled in RCof units and in Factor VIII units. The recommended dosage of Humate or 40–80 IU vWF:RCoF per kg depending on the vWD type and bleeding severity. One vWF:RCoF unit per kg should raise the plasma vWF:RCoF level by 1.5 IU/dL.

Humate P Dosage Guidelines for vWD Based on RCof

vWD Type	Hemorrhage Severity	Loading Dose vWF:RCoF IU/kg	Maintenance Dose vWF:RCoF	Plasma Target Trough Level RCof
1	Minor	40 - 50	40 - 50 q 12h x 1d	
1	Major	40 - 60	40 - 50 q 12h x 3d 40 - 50 q 24h x 4d	RCoF >50%
2 or 3	Minor	40 - 50	40 - 50 x 1	
2 or 3	Major	60 - 80	40 - 60 q 12h x 3d 40 - 60 q 24h x 4d	RCoF >50%

Examples of minor bleeding include epistaxis, oral mucosal bleeding and menorrhagia. Examples of major bleeding include GI, CNS and trauma. If RCoF units are not known, dosage should be based on Factor VIII levels. The recommended dosage based on Factor VIII is 20–40 IU FVIII:C per kgFactor VIII:C Dosage Guidelines for vWD

Humate P Dosage Guidelines Based on Factor VIII:C

Type of Bleeding	FVIII Dose (IU/kg)	Number Infusions	Plasma FVIII:C Target Level (%)
Major Surgery	40 - 60	q 12h day of surgery then once a day	>50 until healing complete
Minor Surgery	30 - 50	Once a day or QOD	>30 until healing complete
Dental Extractions	20 - 30	Single	>30 for one day
Spontaneous bleed	20 - 30	Single	>30

The plasma half life of vWF:RCoF is much shorter than Factor VIII, 8 hours versus 24 hours. Plasma Factor VIII levels should be monitored daily and the dose adjusted accordingly. The patient's plasma Factor VIII level should increase 2U/dL for each 1 IU/kg infused. A patient's own FVIII level will begin to rise within 4 to 8 hours after infusion of vWF.

Factor VIII concentrate is preferred over cryoprecipitate because of the decreased risk of viral transmission. Cryoprecipitate should not be used except in life and limb-threatening emergencies when vWF-containing Factor VIII concentrate is not immediately available. A reasonable dose of cryoprecipitate is 1 bag for every 5 Kg of body weight. This dose should be repeated every 8 to 12 hours. The amount of von Willebrand factor contained within a given unit of cryoprecipitate is highly variable and dependent upon the donor's plasma level. Additional therapeutic intervention is indicated in certain clinical situations. Type 3 patients who continue to bleed and have a prolonged bleeding time should receive platelets.

Pregnancy causes a progressive increase in vWF. Determination of which obstetrical patients will require therapy for delivery should be based on the factor VIII level and not the vWF level. Patients with factor VIII levels >50% usually do not experience increased bleeding with vaginal delivery or C-section. Bleeding can be significant when the Factor VIII level is <20%. A patient with Factor VIII levels <50% should receive DDAVP or Factor VIII concentrate prior to delivery. If prolonged bleeding occurs during delivery, then Factor VIII concentrate should be given regardless of the Factor VIII level. Three to 4 daily doses of Factor VIII concentrate are usually necessary to avoid postpartum bleeding. Pregnant patients with type 2B vWD may develop thrombocytopenia due to increasing vWF levels. Factor concentrate can be given just prior to delivery to reverse thrombocytopenia.

Inhibitors to von Willebrand factor
Repetitive administration of vWF to patients with Type 3 vWD causes alloimmunization in about 15% of patients. Additional doses can cause an anamnestic response. Low level inhibitors can be overwhelmed by administration of high doses.

Pseudo-von Willebrand's disease
Pseudo vWD results from a platelet membrane defect and is not part of the classification of vWD. Platelet membrane glycoprotein Ib has an increased affinity for vWF that causes binding of vWF to platelets and consequent platelet agglutination and thrombocytopenia. DDAVP and Humate P are contraindicated because they can cause a precipitous drop in the platelet count. Patients should be treated with a single donor platelet unit or 6 to 8 random donor platelet concentrates for minor hemorrhages. More severe bleeding may require additional platelet transfusions.

Acquired von Willebrand's Disease (von Willebrand's syndrome)
Diseases or medications that interfere with the function of vWF cause acquired vWD. Diseases include autoimmune disorders, monoclonal gammopathies, lymphoproliferative disorders, adenocarcinoma, squamous cell carcinoma, hepatoma, hypothyroidism, and intestinal telangiectasia. The most commonly associated drug is valproic acid.

Acquired vWD is comparable to Type 1 or 2A vWD. Patients may be either asymptomatic or experience mild to severe hemorrhage. Treatment should be directed at the underlying disease whenever possible. Therapeutic options include DDAVP, Amicar and Humate P. DDAVP has a shortened effect in acquired disease and is contraindicated for patients taking valproic acid because it may precipitate seizures. Antifibrinolytic therapy can be used for oral and nasal mucosal bleeding. Factor concentrates have a shortened half-life and may not be successful.

www.ingramcontent.com/pod-product-compliance
Lightning Source LLC
Chambersburg PA
CBHW081134170526

45165CB00008B/2665